ATLAS OF
LAPAROSCOPIC
UROLOGIC SURGERY

ATLAS OF LAPAROSCOPIC UROLOGIC SURGERY

Jay T. Bishoff, MD

Director
Laparoscopy and Minimally Invasive Surgery Department
Urology San Antonio
San Antonio, Texas

Louis R. Kavoussi, MD

Professor of Urology
New York University School of Medicine
New York, New York
Chairman
The Institute of Urology
North Shore–Long Island Jewish Health System
Manhasset, New York

SAUNDERS

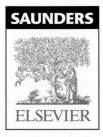

ELSEVIER

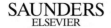

1600 John F. Kennedy Blvd.
Ste 1800
Philadelphia, PA 19103-2899

Atlas of Laparoscopic Urologic Surgery

ISBN-13: 978-1-4160-2580-1
ISBN-10: 1-4160-2580-4

Notice

Knowledge and best practice in this field are constantly changing. As new research and experience broaden our knowledge, changes in practice, treatment and drug therapy may become necessary or appropriate. Readers are advised to check the most current information provided (i) on procedures featured or (ii) by the manufacturer of each product to be administered, to verify the recommended dose or formula, the method and duration of administration, and contraindications. It is the responsibility of the practitioner, relying on their own experience and knowledge of the patient, to make diagnoses, to determine dosages and the best treatment for each individual patient, and to take all appropriate safety precautions. To the fullest extent of the law, neither the Publisher nor the Editors/Authors assumes any liability for any injury and/or damage to persons or property arising out or related to any use of the material contained in this book.

The Publisher

Library of Congress Cataloging-in-Publication Data
Atlas of laparoscopic urologic surgery / [edited by] Jay T. Bishoff, Louis R. Kavoussi.—1st ed.
    p. ; cm.
   Includes bibliographical references.
   ISBN 1-4160-2580-4
  1. Endourology—Atlases. I. Bishoff, Jay T. II. Kavoussi, Louis R.
   [DNLM: 1. Laparoscopy—methods—Atlases. 2. Urologic Surgical Procedures—methods—Atlases. WJ 17 A88155 2007]

RD572.A85 2007
617.4′60597—dc22

                                 2006031894

Acquisitions Editor: Rebecca Gaertner
Editorial Assistant: Suzanne Flint
Publishing Services Manager: Tina Rebane
Project Manager: Amy L. Cannon
Design Director: Karen O'Keefe Owens

Printed in China

Last digit is the print number: 9 8 7 6 5 4 3 2 1

A surgeon's life is never his or her own. Patient care has a vested interest in our lives and extracts its share, often at inopportune and inconvenient times. As a result, we dedicate this book to surgeons' families for their love, support, and tolerance of our life's work.

CLEMENT-CLAUDE ABBOU, MD
Professor and Chief, Service d'Urologie Centre Hospitalier
Universitaire Henri Mondor, Créteil, France
Laparoscopic Prostatectomy: Preperitoneal Approach

MOHAMAD E. ALLAF, MD
Assistant Professor of Urology, The James Buchanan Brady
Urological Institute, The Johns Hopkins Hospital, Baltimore,
Maryland
Laparoscopic Retroperitoneal Lymph Node Dissection

J. KYLE ANDERSON, MD
Department of Urologic Surgery, University of Minnesota,
Minneapolis, Minnesota
Laparoscopic Radical Nephrectomy

TIMOTHY D. AVERCH, MD
Assistant Professor and Director of Endourology, Department
of Urology, University of Pittsburgh Medical Center,
Pittsburgh, Pennsylvania
Laparoscopic Simple Nephrectomy

D. DUANE BALDWIN, MD
Associate Professor, Division of Urology, Loma Linda
University Medical Center, Loma Linda, California
Laparoscopic Pelvic Lymph Node Dissection

ADAM J. BALL, MD
Endourology/Laparoscopy Fellow, Devine-Tidewater Urology,
Sentara Norfolk General Hospital, Eastern Virginia Medical
School, Norfolk, Virginia
Laparoscopic Donor Nephrectomy

STEVEN M. BAUGHMAN, MD
Chief Resident, Urology, Department of Urology, Wilford
Hall Medical Center, Lackland Air Force Base, San Antonio,
Texas
Laparoscopic Orchiopexy

SAM B. BHAYANI, MD
Assistant Professor, Division of Urologic Surgery, Washington
University School of Medicine, Saint Louis, Missouri
Laparoscopic Pyeloplasty

JAY T. BISHOFF, MD
Director, Laparoscopy and Minimally Invasive Surgery
Department, Urology San Antonio, San Antonio, Texas
*Basic Techniques in Laparoscopic Surgery; Endoscopic Subcutaneous Modified
Inguinal Lymph Node Dissection for Squamous Cell Carcinoma of the Penis*

MAJ IAN H. BLACK, MD, MC
Assistant Professor of Anesthesiology, Uniformed Services
University of the Health Sciences; Director, TARGIT Center;
Chief of Anesthesia, United States Army Institute of Surgical
Research, Fort Sam Houston, Texas
Anesthetic Implications of Minimally Invasive Urologic Surgery

JEFFREY A. CADEDDU, MD
Associate Professor of Urology and Director, Clinical Center
for Minimally Invasive Urologic Cancer Treatment,
Department of Urology, The University of Texas
Southwestern Medical Center, Dallas, Texas
Laparoscopic Radical Nephrectomy

EARL Y. CHENG, MD
Associate Professor, Department of Urology, Northwestern
University Feinberg School of Medicine; Attending Urologist,
Department of Urology, Children's Memorial Hospital,
Chicago, Illinois
Laparoscopic Orchiopexy

GEORGE K. CHOW, MD
Assistant Professor, Mayo Clinic College of Medicine;
Department of Urology, Mayo Clinic, Rochester, Minnesota
Hand-Assisted Laparoscopic Radical Nephrectomy

CHARALAMBOS DELIVELIOTIS, MD, PhD
Associate Professor, Second Department of Urology,
University of Athens School of Medicine, Sismanoglio
Hospital, Athens, Greece
Laparoscopic Ureterolithotomy

PREMAL J. DESAI, MD
Resident Physician, Division of Urology, Loma Linda
University Medical Center, Loma Linda, California
Laparoscopic Pelvic Lymph Node Dissection

STEVEN G. DOCIMO, MD
Professor of Urology and Director, Pediatric Urology, The
Children's Hospital of Pittsburgh; Vice Chairman,
Department of Urology, The University of Pittsburgh
Medical Center, Pittsburgh, Pennsylvania
Pediatric Laparoscopic Pyeloplasty

DAVID A. DUCHENE, MD
Endourology Fellow, Department of Urology, The University
of Kansas, Kansas City, Kansas
Laparoscopic Radical Nephrectomy

LARS ELLISON, MD
Director of Laparoscopic Urologic Surgery Program and
Assistant Professor, Department of Urology, University of
California, Davis, Sacramento, California
Laparoscopic Ureterolysis and Repair of Retrocaval Ureter

MICHAEL D. FABRIZIO, MD
Associate Professor of Urology, Urology of Virginia, Sentara
Norfolk General Hospital, Eastern Virginia Medical School,
Norfolk, Virginia
*Laparoscopic Donor Nephrectomy; Laparoscopic Evaluation and Treatment of
Symptomatic and Indeterminate Renal Cysts*

MATTHEW T. GETTMAN, MD
Associate Professor, Department of Urology, Mayo Clinic
College of Medicine, Rochester, Minnesota
Laparoscopic Prostatectomy: Preperitoneal Approach

**KURT W. GRATHWOHL, MD, FCCP, LTC,
USA, MC**
Assistant Professor of Medicine and Anesthesiology,
Uniformed Services University of the Health Sciences,
Bethesda, Maryland; Associate Professor of Surgery, Division
of Trauma, University of Texas Health Sciences Center, San
Antonio, Texas; Chief, Division of Anesthesia/Critical Care,
Department of Anesthesia and Operative Services, Brooke
Army Medical Center, Fort Sam Houston, Texas
Anesthetic Implications of Minimally Invasive Urologic Surgery

BLAKE D. HAMILTON, MD
Associate Professor, Division of Urology, University of Utah
School of Medicine, Salt Lake City, Utah
Laparoscopic Adrenalectomy

SEAN P. HEDICAN, MD
Associate Professor, Department of Urology, University of
Wisconsin Medical School, Madison, Wisconsin
Hand-Assisted Laparoscopic Radical Nephroureterectomy

ANDRÁS HOZNEK, MD
Service d'Urologie, Centre Hospitalier Universitaire Henri
Mondor, Créteil, France
Laparoscopic Prostatectomy: Preperitoneal Approach

STEPHEN V. JACKMAN, MD
Associate Professor, Department of Urology, University of
Pittsburgh Medical Center, Pittsburgh, Pennsylvania
Laparoscopic Renal Biopsy

THOMAS W. JARRETT, MD
Professor and Chairman of Urology, The George Washington
University, Washington, DC
Laparoscopic Nephroureterectomy

LOUIS R. KAVOUSSI, MD
Professor of Urology, New York University School of
Medicine, New York; Chairman, The Institute of Urology,
North Shore–Long Island Jewish Health System, Manhasset,
New York
Complications of Laparoscopic Surgery

JAIME LANDMAN, MD
Assistant Professor, Department of Urology, Columbia
University School of Medicine, New York, New York
Laparoscopic and Percutaneous Delivery of Renal Ablative Technology

BENJAMIN R. LEE, MD
Associate Professor, Department of Urology, Long Island
Jewish Medical Center, New Hyde Park, New York
Closure Techniques and Exiting the Abdomen

DAVID I. LEE, MD
Assistant Professor of Surgery/Urology, University of
Pennsylvania School of Medicine; Chief of Urology, Penn
Presbyterian Medical Center, Philadelphia, Pennsylvania
Robotic Prostatectomy

CLAUDIO MONTIOLA, MD
Urologist, Hospital Clinico de la Fuerza Aerea de Chile,
Santiago, Chile
*Endoscopic Subcutaneous Modified Inguinal Lymph Node Dissection for
Squamous Cell Carcinoma of the Penis*

STEPHEN Y. NAKADA, MD
Chairman, Division of Urology, Department of Surgery and
The David T. Uehling Professor of Urology, University of
Wisconsin–Madison Medical School, Madison, Wisconsin
Laparoscopic Stapling and Reconstruction

MIKE NGUYEN, MD
Resident, Department of Urology, University of California,
Davis, Sacramento, California
Laparoscopic Ureterolysis and Repair of Retrocaval Ureter

PAUL H. NOH, MD
Assistant Professor of Urology and Pediatrics, Thomas
Jefferson University, Jefferson Medical College, Philadelphia,
Pennsylvania; Staff Urologist, Division of Urology,
Department of Surgery, Alfred I. duPont Hospital for
Children, Wilmington, Delaware
Pediatric Laparoscopic Pyeloplasty

GYAN PAREEK, MD
Assistant Professor of Surgery, Division of Urology, Brown
Medical School, Providence, Rhode Island
Laparoscopic Stapling and Reconstruction

CHRISTIAN P. PAVLOVICH, MD

Associate Professor, Brady Urological Institute, Johns Hopkins Medical Institutions; Director, Urologic Oncology, Johns Hopkins Bayview Medical Center, Department of Urology, Baltimore, Maryland
Laparoscopic Radical Cystectomy and Urinary Diversion

PETER A. PINTO, MD

Senior Investigator, Urologic Oncology Branch, National Cancer Institute, National Institutes of Health, Bethesda, Maryland
Laparoscopic Partial Nephrectomy

KOON HO RHA, MD, PhD

Assistant Professor, Department of Urology, Yonsei University College of Medicine, Seoul, Korea
Laparoscopic Ureteral Reimplantation and Boari Flap

DANIEL J. RICCHIUTI, MD

Assistant Professor in Urology, Northeastern Ohio Universities College of Medicine, Rootstown, Ohio
Laparoscopic Simple Nephrectomy

LEE RICHSTONE, MD

Attending Physician, Department of Urology, The Institute of Urology, North Shore–Long Island Jewish Health System, Manhasset, New York
Complications of Laparoscopic Surgery

WILLIAM W. ROBERTS, MD

Assistant Professor, Department of Urology, University of Michigan Health System, Ann Arbor, Michigan
Hand-Assisted Laparoscopic Radical Nephroureterectomy

EDWIN L. ROBEY, MD

Associate Professor of Urology, Devine-Tidewater Urology, Sentara Norfolk General Hospital, Eastern Virginia Medical School, Norfolk, Virginia
Laparoscopic Donor Nephrectomy

LAURENT SALOMON, MD, PhD

Deparmente of Urology, Paris XII Faculty; Service d'Urologie, Henri Mondor Hospital, Créteil, France
Laparoscopic Prostatectomy: Preperitoneal Approach

C. WILLIAM SCHWAB II, MD

Instructor of Urology, Eastern Virginia Medical School, Norfolk, Virginia
Laparoscopic Nephroureterectomy

PHILIPPE SÈBE, MD, PhD

Lecturer, Department of Anatomy, Pierre and Marie Curie University; Surgeon, Department of Urology, Tenon Hospital, Paris, France
Laparoscopic Prostatectomy: Preperitoneal Approach

DOUG W. SODERDAHL, MD, LT COL, USA, MC

Department of Urology, Brooke Army Medical Center, Fort Sam Houston, Texas
Laparoscopic Evaluation and Treatment of Symptomatic and Indeterminate Renal Cysts

LI-MING SU, MD

Associate Professor of Urology and Director of Laparoscopy and Robotic Urologic Surgery, James Buchanan Brady Urological Institute, Johns Hopkins Medical Institutions, Baltimore, Maryland
Nerve-Sparing Laparoscopic Radical Prostatectomy: Transperitoneal Technique

ITAY Y. VARDI, MD

Fellow in Laparoscopy, Department of Surgery, Washington University School of Medicine, Saint Louis, Missouri
Laparoscopic Pyeloplasty

IOANNIS VARKARAKIS, MD, PhD

Lecturer in Urology, Second Department of Urology, University of Athens School of Medicine, Sismanoglio Hospital, Athens, Greece
Laparoscopic Ureterolithotomy

ANDREW A. WAGNER, MD

Assistant Professor, Harvard Medical School, Boston, Massachusetts
Laparoscopic Radical Cystectomy and Urinary Diversion

KYLE J. WELD, MD

Minimally Invasive Urology Fellow, Division of Urology, Washington University School of Medicine, Saint Louis, Missouri
Laparoscopic and Percutaneous Delivery of Renal Ablative Technology

CHRISTOPHER R. WILLIAMS, MD

Urologic Oncology Fellow, Urologic Oncology Branch, National Cancer Institute, National Institutes of Health, Bethesda, Maryland
Laparoscopic Partial Nephrectomy

ELIZABETH B. YERKES, MD

Assistant Professor of Urology, Department of Urology, Northwestern University Feinberg School of Medicine; Attending Urologist, Department of Urology, Children's Memorial Hospital, Chicago, Illinois
Laparoscopic Orchiopexy

CONTENTS

That which we persist in doing becomes easier, not that the task itself has become easier,
but that our ability to perform it has improved.

Ralph Waldo Emerson
1803–1882

Since Bill Schuessler's first transperitoneal endosurgical lymphadenectomy in a patient with localized prostate cancer (performed in October 1989), urologists have slowly accepted the forces of change, leading them away from the traditions of open surgical approaches toward minimally invasive routes to treat operative pathology. This transition has been fueled by creative surgeons and by an increasingly educated patient population seeking less morbid treatment for diseases. The combination of changes has lead to a surgical revolution, with the patient being the ultimate beneficiary. Before these changes can become widely available, surgeons must gain the ability to perform new techniques. The process of learning a completely new operative technique is uncomfortable for the surgeon, who recognizes the benefits for the patient and of trying to gain the ability to perform a new task. This atlas was created to help ease the pain in the process of gaining new "abilities" or surgical skills.

Our first text, *The Atlas of Laparoscopic Retroperitoneal Surgery*, published in 2000, was well received, but in a very short time became outdated, mainly due to the absence of many new laparoscopic procedures that have passed through the appropriate filters of criticism and scientific scrutiny. Our second text, *The Atlas of Laparoscopic Urologic Surgery*, has a new name that more accurately describes the scope of the text and covers the most current laparoscopic urologic procedures. The goal of this new project remains the same as the first; introduce surgeons to the use of laparoscopy in the treatment of urologic disease by providing detailed descriptions of basic techniques, anesthesia considerations, surgical procedures, and treatment of complications in order to shorten the learning curve associated with initial applications of new procedures and learning new surgical skills. We appreciate the contributions by various experts from busy laparoscopic centers who have taken time from their practices to share their experiences in different operative techniques learned through repetition, mistakes, and perseverance.

This text begins with a description of basic instrumentation and techniques. Anesthesia considerations unique to laparoscopic surgery are detailed in a separate chapter written by anesthesiologists and pulmonary critical care experts. The chapters that follow detail specific surgical procedures and are structured to discuss potential applications as well as contraindications. As each technique is described, attention is given to patient positioning and port placement. Detailed line drawings were created from the perspective of the laparoscope, compliment the point-by-point instruction given in the text, and demonstrate critical steps for each procedure. Where differences exist between left and right approaches, thorough, contrasting descriptions and diagrams are provided. Each chapter ends with recommended postoperative management strategies and at least one Tips and Tricks Box. The book concludes with a detailed discussion of the recognition and treatment of laparoscopic complications.

We are happy to include a DVD with this edition of *The Atlas of Laparoscopic Urologic Surgery*. Many important steps for selected procedures are included in the DVD, contributed by the respective authors of the pertinent chapters. The companion DVD covers important surgical steps to help the surgeon grasp the surgical and anatomic concepts of the procedure.

The production of a detailed atlas of this type requires significant efforts from many individuals. We would like to thank all of the contributors for their timely and complete contributions. We want to recognize the artistic talents of Nancy Place, whose beautiful line drawings unify the atlas and add the detail necessary to understand the procedures described in each chapter. We are indebted to her for her dedication to this project. Finally, we would like to express our gratitude to Elsevier and in particular Rebecca Gaertner, Suzanne Flint, and Amy Cannon for their guidance and patience in producing this text.

JAY T. BISHOFF, MD
LOUIS R. KAVOUSSI, MD

CHAPTER 1

Basic Techniques in Laparoscopic Surgery

Jay T. Bishoff

Techniques in laparoscopic surgery have evolved greatly over the past several years. Presently, only the surgeon's imagination and the industry's willingness to produce innovative equipment limit the future development of new laparoscopic equipment. In this chapter, state-of-the-art methods for insufflation, access, dissection, hemostasis, retraction, tissue retrieval, robotic camera assistance, and intraoperative imaging are presented. The goal of the chapter is to increase the surgeon's repertoire of techniques in order to condense the learning curve, shorten procedure times, and improve patient outcomes. The final section in this chapter describes the indications and technique of retroperitoneal access. Separate chapters in this atlas are dedicated to reconstruction (including suturing and stapling), closure of the abdomen, and complications.

INSUFFLATION

Inspect the insufflator before the start of the case to ensure proper function, and check the CO_2 cylinder to ensure an adequate quantity of gas. From experience I have found that if there is insufficient CO_2 to complete the procedure, it will usually run empty at the most crucial part of the operation. Circulating nurses in the operating room must be familiar with the procedure of changing the CO_2 tank, and a spare tank must be available in the room at the start of the procedure. Attach sterile tubing at the beginning of the case, and check the pressure-flow mechanism by turning the gas flow to high and occluding the tubing. A rapid increase in pressure, above the preset limit, should cause flow of gas to cease. Then set initial pressure on the machine at 15 to 20 mm Hg.

PNEUMOPERITONEUM

It is my practice to create a pneumoperitoneum with the Veress needle before placing the first trocar. This simple technique is essentially unchanged since 1991 and is applicable to almost every laparoscopic situation. The pneumoperitoneum is accomplished by blindly passing the Veress needle into the peritoneum. The retracting tip and small size of the Veress needle help to minimize the risk of injury to underlying structures (Fig. 1–1).

In those patients without prior abdominal midline incisions, the umbilicus is a good site for initial entry with the Veress needle and the first trocar. At the umbilicus, the fascial layers fuse together allowing rapid entry into the peritoneum, the peritoneum is closer to the skin, and the incision is well concealed in this region (Fig. 1–2). Place a stay suture, if needed, at the site of initial entry to help elevate the abdominal wall and secure the trocar once in place. Holding the Veress needle like a dart, pass the tip perpendicular to the abdominal wall. Typically, two distinct layers are passed with the needle and then the blunt core pops forward: the first layer is the fascia, and the second is the peritoneum.

When the needle has advanced into the peritoneum, attach a 10-mL syringe containing 5 mL of normal saline to the needle. First, perform aspiration to detect any return of blood or bowel contents, which would require removal of the needle, replacement at a different site, and careful inspection of the underlying structures once the laparoscope is introduced into the abdomen. After aspiration, pass at least 5 mL of saline into the abdominal cavity, and attempt aspiration again. If the peritoneal cavity has been entered, saline usually will not return to the syringe with aspiration. If there is a return of saline, the needle is usually in the preperitoneal space and must be repositioned before attempting insufflation. Finally, after removing the syringe from the Veress needle, a small amount of saline will be seen in the hub of the needle where it was connected to the syringe. Correct placement of the needle allows any fluid left in the needle to fall into the abdomen once the syringe is disconnected.

Once the needle placement has passed all of these tests, attach the insufflation tubing to the needle and initially set the flow of gas at 1 L/min. The initial patient pressure needs to be less than 10 mm Hg, with the needle in the peritoneal cavity and the insufflator set on low flow. Higher pressures may indicate improper placement of the needle or occlusion of the tip of the needle against the bowel wall. If the pressure is greater than 10 mm Hg, elevate the abdominal wall and turn or retract the needle. If an elevated pressure reading persists, withdraw the needle immediately (before 150 mL of gas has been instilled). It will be necessary to pass the needle again, repeating all of the prior steps. If even a moderate amount of CO_2 gas is instilled in the preperitoneal space, it will be very difficult to gain access and have the trocar in the correct position during the procedure. If it appears that the needle was preperitoneal, the surgeon needs to move away from the initial site for repeat attempts at placement of the Veress needle.

As the peritoneal cavity fills with gas, there should be symmetrical expansion and loss of the dullness to percussion replaced with tympani. If there is asymmetric distention of the abdomen, the needle is probably not in correct position and a

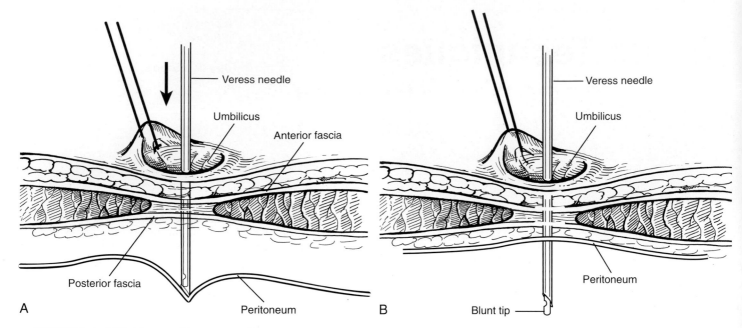

FIGURE 1–1. *A,* The blunt tip of the Veress needle retracts as it comes in contact with the skin, allowing the sharp needle to penetrate skin, fascia, and perito-neum. *B,* When the needle enters the empty space of the abdominal cavity, the blunt tip springs forward protecting underlying abdominal structures from injury. The sound of the blunt tip springing forward helps alert the surgeon that the abdominal cavity has been entered.

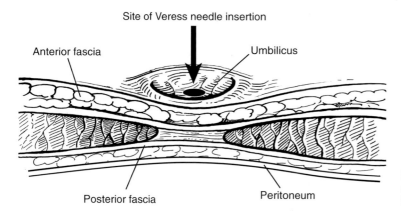

FIGURE 1–2. In patients without prior abdominal surgery through a midline incision, the umbilicus is an excellent site of entry. The incision is well concealed and the peritoneum is close to the skin.

new site, some distance away from the first site, needs to be chosen for needle placement (Fig. 1–3).

After instilling 1 to 1.5 L of gas into the abdomen and not detecting elevated pressures, turn the flow from the insufflator to high, even though the maximum flow through a Veress needle is less than 3 L/min. Approximately 4 to 6 L of gas will be required to completely distend the abdomen to a pressure of 15 to 20 mm Hg.

In patients with a history of abdominal surgery, pass the Veress needle and initial trocar at a site far from the previous incision sites. Avoid insertion over the liver, spleen, and left lower quadrant (where adhesion may be present from episodes of diverticulitis) if possible (Fig. 1–4).

CO_2 is the gas most commonly used for insufflation during laparoscopic surgery. It has the properties of high blood solubil-ity and rapid absorption and does not support combustion. Although CO_2 is absorbed in the blood, it is removed in the lung during exhalation. A fatal intravascular dose of CO_2 in animals is five times greater than a fatal dose of room air (25 mL/kg CO_2 versus 5 mL/kg air).[1] Sudden cardiovascular

collapse during laparoscopy may be secondary to gas embo-lism from needle placement into a blood vessel or highly vascular organ. Once a large volume of air enters the vascular system, the gas can accumulate in the right ventricle, obstruct-ing the pulmonary blood flow and leading to cardiovascular collapse. The treatment is to immediately decompress the peri-toneum and place the patient into the right-side-up, left-side-down, head-down position (Durant position). This position allows the gas to rise and blood flow through the right heart to continue (Fig. 1–5). In addition, start ventilation with 100% oxygen.

An initial insufflation pressure of 20 mm Hg creates a full and tense abdomen, facilitating trocar placement. This pressure is also helpful in maintaining an adequate pneumo-peritoneum and working space because gas will escape during the procedure through and around trocar sites. Often, the obese patient requires a working pressure of 20 mm Hg during the entire case. In other patients, the pressure can usually be decreased to 10 to 15 mm Hg for the duration of the case. I try to work at the lowest pressure possible, given the

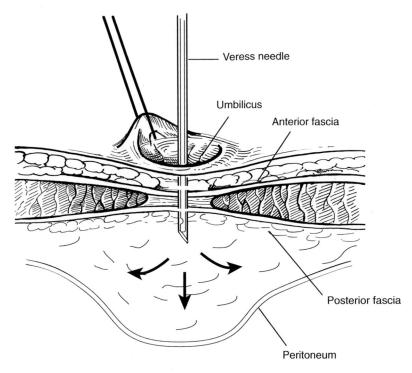

FIGURE 1–3. As the abdominal cavity fills with gas there should be symmetrical expansion and loss of the dullness to percussion. If there is asymmetric distension of the abdomen, the needle may be in the preperitoneal space. A different site, away from the first, should be chosen for needle placement.

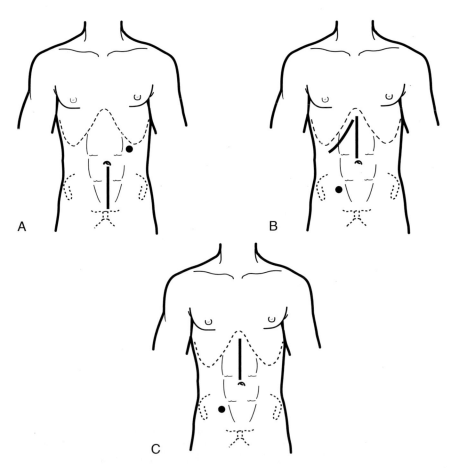

FIGURE 1–4. Sites of Veress needle placement for insufflation and initial trocar placement in patients who have undergone prior abdominal surgery.

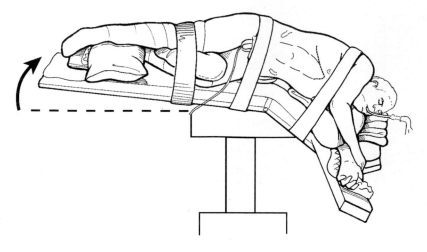

FIGURE 1–5. Sudden cardiovascular collapse from a pulmonary gas embolism is treated by immediate decompression of the pneumoperitoneum and placement of the patient in the right-side-elevated, head-down position.

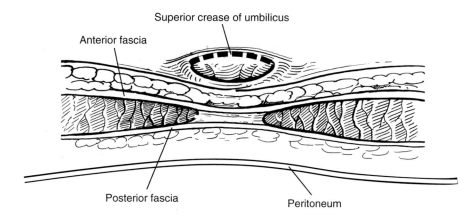

FIGURE 1–6. A curvilinear incision in the umbilicus is well concealed and offers excellent cosmesis.

patient's anatomy and the area of dissection, that will allow adequate visualization.

Adverse physiologic changes are seen at high abdominal pressures. As the intra-abdominal pressure is gradually increased above 25 mm Hg, there is decreased venous return to the heart. At pressures greater than 30 mm Hg, there is a decrease in cardiac output and hypotension may occur.[2]

The respiratory effects of pneumoperitoneum can be significant, particularly in patients with preexisting cardiopulmonary disease who manifest increased end-tidal CO_2, increased arterial CO_2, decreased arterial pH, higher peak airway pressure, and increased minute ventilation.[3] Increased ventilating volume and pressure may worsen the risk of barotrauma and pneumothorax in these patients. Healthy patients, on the other hand, demonstrate a mild increase in end-tidal CO_2 and arterial CO_2, a decrease in arterial pH, but no significant changes in peak airway pressure or minute volume[4] (see Chapter 3, Anesthetic Implications of Minimally Invasive Urologic Surgery).

TROCAR PLACEMENT

Primary Trocar

Site Selection

Place the first trocar in the same site as the Veress needle insertion for insufflation. In many cases, the umbilicus is the site of choice. A curvilinear incision made at the umbilicus after insuf-

flation is well concealed and offers an excellent cosmetic result (Fig. 1–6). When patients are in complete lateral or a modified lateral position, a site lateral to the rectus muscle may be the best site for initial insufflation and trocar placement because bowel may have moved closer to the umbilicus. After placing the lateral trocar, place the remaining ports under direct visualization. During placement, direct all trocars slightly toward the area of surgical interest to allow decreased tension during dissection and to help prevent trocar site holes from being aligned. Staggering the access site from entry at a slight angle will decrease the chance for hernia formation (Fig. 1–7).

Visual Obturator

After insufflation, place the initial port under direct vision using a trocar with a visual obturator. When using a visual obturator, turn the light source to low, and place the laparoscope inside the visual obturator, focusing on the clear lens, and through the initial trocar sheath. With either gentle twisting motion or a trigger mechanism, divide the muscle and peritoneum under direct vision.

Several trocars with a visual obturator are currently available and allow access under direct vision. The 12-mm Visiport Plus RPF trocar (U.S. Surgical, Norwalk, CT) uses a recessed blade that extends out of the end of the obturator as the surgeon fires a trigger on the pistol grip (Fig. 1–8). The newly engineered Endopath Xcel trocar (Ethicon Endo-Surgery, Cincinnati, OH) and the Optical Separator (Applied Medical, Rancho

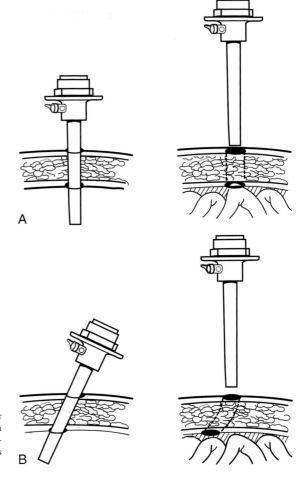

FIGURE 1–7. *A,* A trocar placed directly perpendicular to the fascia can allow the anterior and posterior fascial entry sites to line up after the trocar is removed and will be under tension during the dissection. *B,* A trocar placed at a slight angle directed toward the site of dissection will leave the anterior and posterior entry sites staggered and allow dissection with less tension on the skin.

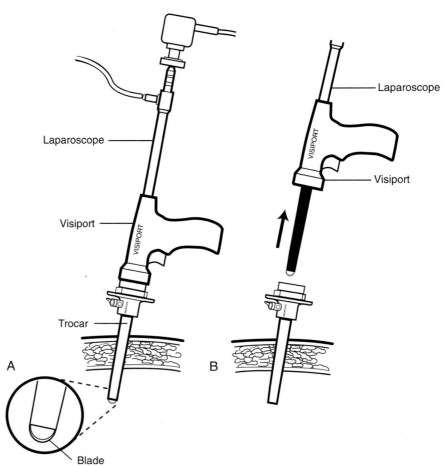

FIGURE 1–8. *A,* The Visiport Plus RPF trocar (U.S. Surgical, Norwalk, CT) uses a recessed blade that extends out of the end of the obturator as the surgeon fires a trigger to incise fascia, muscle, and peritoneum under direct vision. *B,* Once the trocar is in the abdominal cavity, the Visiport is removed.

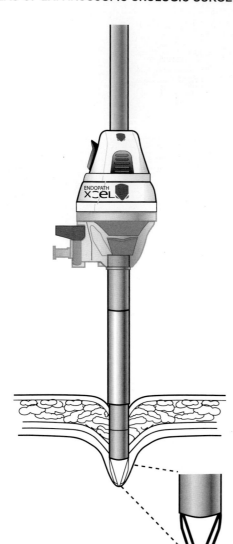

FIGURE 1–9. The Endopath Xcel trocar (Ethicon Endo-Surgery, Inc., Cincinnati, OH) system uses two sharpened blades on the tip of the trocar. A gentle twisting motion uses the blades to cut through the abdominal layers into the peritoneum under direct vision.

Santa Margarita, CA) 12-mm and 5-mm systems use two sharpened ridges (in different configurations) on the tip of the trocar to divide fascia and enter the peritoneum, while the surgeon watches via the laparoscope inserted through the center of the trocar (Fig. 1–9). These systems allow rapid entry under direct vision, with potentially less risk of injury compared with blind trocar insertion.

Hasson Cannula

The Hasson technique of initial port placement may be useful for patients with a history of extensive or multiple abdominal surgeries or peritonitis. The Hasson system consists of a trumpet valve with tying struts, cone-shaped sleeve, and blunt-tipped obturator. Make a 2- to 3-cm incision in the skin at the insertion site, sweep the preperitoneal fat off the fascia, and incise the fascia. Elevate the peritoneum with a pair of forceps and open it sharply. Confirm entry into the peritoneal cavity by looking directly or by passing the index finger into the perito-

neal cavity. Place two 0 monofilament fascial stay sutures, and include the edge of the peritoneum. These sutures can be used at the end of the case to close the trocar site. Insert the Hasson system through the peritonotomy and push down the conical collar into the skin incision to occlude the opening, preventing escape of CO_2 during insufflation. The fascial sutures secure the trocar to the abdomen and help to keep the cone-shaped collar seated. Attach the insufflation tubing and create the pneumoperitoneum.

Place the AutoSuture Blunt Tip Trocar (U.S. Surgical, Norwalk, CT) in fashion similar to the traditional Hasson trocar, that is, through a small open incision. This trocar uses an inflated balloon on the inside and a locking foam collar on the skin to create an airtight seal. The cap allows use of 5-mm, 10-mm, and 12-mm instruments and has insufflation and desufflation ports. The low profile of the trocar makes it especially useful for working in the limited space of the retroperitoneum (Fig. 1–10).

Secondary Trocar

After placing the primary trocar, insert a laparoscope into the abdomen and perform a thorough survey, looking for any evidence of injury, adhesions, or unexpected pathology during Veress needle and primary trocar placement. Place all secondary trocars under direct vision. The exact position of trocar placement is dependent on the procedure being performed and experience with the laparoscopic procedure. Trocars that are placed too close together make it difficult to dissect in the abdomen and limit movement because handles and trocars collide.

Before placing a trocar, use a finger to indent the outside of the abdominal wall at the purposed trocar site. While looking from the purposed site to the area of dissection (using the view from inside the abdomen), make adjustments before committing to a particular site. Remove adhesions near proposed trocar sites before placing the trocar in order to avoid injury to the bowel during trocar placement or during closure. If desired, place a long spinal needle at the proposed trocar site into the abdomen as a so-called finder needle to further identify the exact location inside the abdomen. Recommended sites for trocar placement are carefully described and diagrammed in the chapters of this atlas for each specific procedure.

After determining the trocar site, direct the laparoscope so that the skin is transilluminated, identifying blood vessels and the rectus muscles to avoid during trocar placement. In particular, the large inferior epigastric vessels can usually be identified with transillumination and injury avoided.

Create a skin incision at the trocar site with a No. 11 blade, and use a hemostat to spread the subcutaneous tissue to the level of the fascia. Do not create an incision that is too large because this will result in continual escape of CO_2 during the procedure and may lead to subcutaneous emphysema, acidosis, or even a pneumothorax and pneumomediastinum due to communication with the subcutaneous space. Make the incision just large enough to allow the obturator and the trocar sheath to enter the skin. An incision that is too small will not allow the trocar under the skin and puts the underlying structures at risk for perforation because excess force is required to enter the abdomen and, if the trocar suddenly gives way during insertion, the trocar may not be able to be stopped and it may damage bowel, other organs, or major vessels.

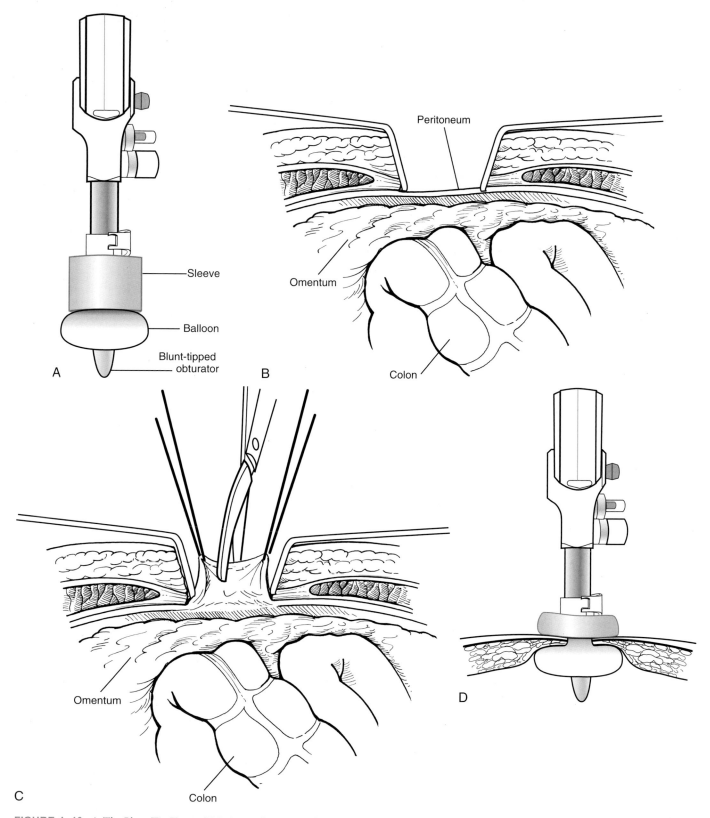

FIGURE 1–10. *A,* The Blunt Tip Trocar (U.S. Surgical) consists of a balloon inflated inside the working space and a locking foam sleeve that creates a gas tight seal. *B,* A 2- to 3-cm incision is made in the skin at the insertion site, the subcutaneous fat swept off the fascia, and the fascia incised. *C,* The peritoneum is elevated and opened sharply. Entry into the peritoneal cavity is confirmed with direct vision or by passing the index finger into the peritoneal cavity. *D,* The trocar is inserted into the cavity, the balloon filled with air, and the foam sleeve slid down onto the skin and locked in place to prevent escape of CO_2 during insufflation.

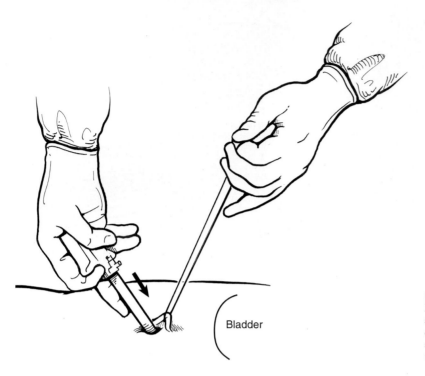

Bladder

FIGURE 1–11. During trocar placement, grasping the skin or lifting the stay suture to apply counter traction elevates the abdominal wall. The surgeon holds the trocar firmly in the dominant hand, with one finger extended along the sheath to act as a brake. A gentle constant twisting motion will help the trocar advance.

During secondary trocar placement, move the insufflation port on the trocar to the closed position to prevent rapid escape of insufflate during placement. Grasp the trocar firmly in the dominant hand, with one finger extended along the sheath to act as brake. Use a gentle constant twisting motion slightly toward the area of dissection to help the trocar advance (Fig. 1–11). Carefully watch the tip of the trocar under direct vision with the laparoscope. Direct the trocar slightly toward the area of dissection while advancing into the peritoneal space (Fig. 1–12). If the trocar is advanced in a direction away from the site of dissection, there will be constant tension on the skin during the case, tension on instruments when not in use, and increased chance for gas to escape at the trocar site. Once the trocar is in place, position it so that approximately 1.5 cm of the trocar is inside the peritoneal cavity. Place a suture through the skin and wrap each strand around the insufflation port (Fig. 1–13) so that the trocar can easily be advanced if necessary and pulled back to the limit of the suture without being inadvertently pulled out of the abdomen during stapling or suturing (Fig. 1–14).

Occasionally, even an experienced surgeon creates a skin entry site that is too large for the trocar, allowing CO_2 to escape. Several steps can be taken to narrow the opening or prevent subcutaneous emphysema and loss of intra-abdominal pressure during the procedure. Try placing a skin suture or penetrating towel clamp to narrow the skin opening and stop gas escaping. In addition, try wrapping a gauze sponge coated with petroleum jelly around the trocar and pushing the sponge against the skin to seal the site.

Inspect all trocar sites for bleeding with the laparoscope after insertion. Persistent bleeding from a lateral trocar site or hematoma formation may indicate injury to the rectus muscle or laceration of the inferior epigastric vessels. Slow oozing from a site will usually stop shortly after port placement due to the tamponade effect of the trocar. Treat sites that have persistent bleeding with a figure-of-eight suture passed on a straight needle above and below the site and secured on the abdomen (Fig. 1–15).

DISSECTION

Safe dissection during laparoscopy requires knowledge of the characteristics and location of tissue planes. With blunt and sharp dissection, these planes can be exploited to expose the desired structures and organs with little trauma and minimal bleeding. Each laparoscopic surgeon has a preference regarding instruments used for dissection. Many use a combination of scissors with monopolar electrocautery, bipolar electrocautery, ultrasonic (US) energy, and blunt dissection with the tip of the irrigator aspirator. Others prefer to use a hook electrode. The tip of the irrigator aspirator is useful as a blunt instrument during dissection. The tissue can be trapped with the tip while applying suction and then spread in the opposite direction of a grasper to open a tissue plane; then the suction is discontinued and the tissue is released (Fig. 1–16).

HYDRODISSECTION

Waterjet cutting and hydrodissection continue to be areas of active investigation for lymph node dissection and partial nephrectomy. Hydrodissection is advanced technology using water at high pressure to act as a sharp instrument. In the past it has been used in delicate corneal surgery and cholecystectomy. In laparoscopic partial nephrectomy, a hydrojet generator (Muritz 1000; Euromed Medizintechnik, Schermwin, Germany) has been used to create a thin stream of water under great pressure (30 atm) that rapidly separates renal parenchyma while preserving vasculature, which can be coagulated and divided using conventional cautery.[5]

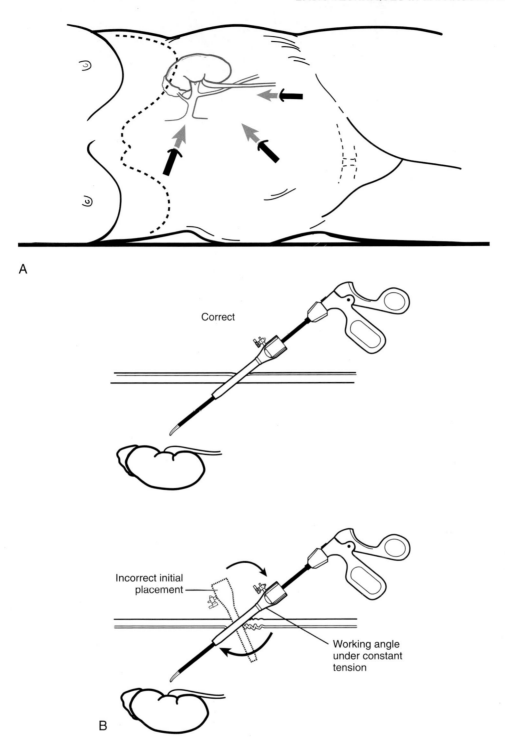

FIGURE 1–12. *A*, The trocar should be directed slightly toward the area of dissection as it is advanced into the abdominal cavity. *B*, Placement of the trocar at a correct angle allows dissection without tension on the instrument. If the trocar is inserted at an angle away from the site of dissection, there will be constant tension on the instrument and trocar.

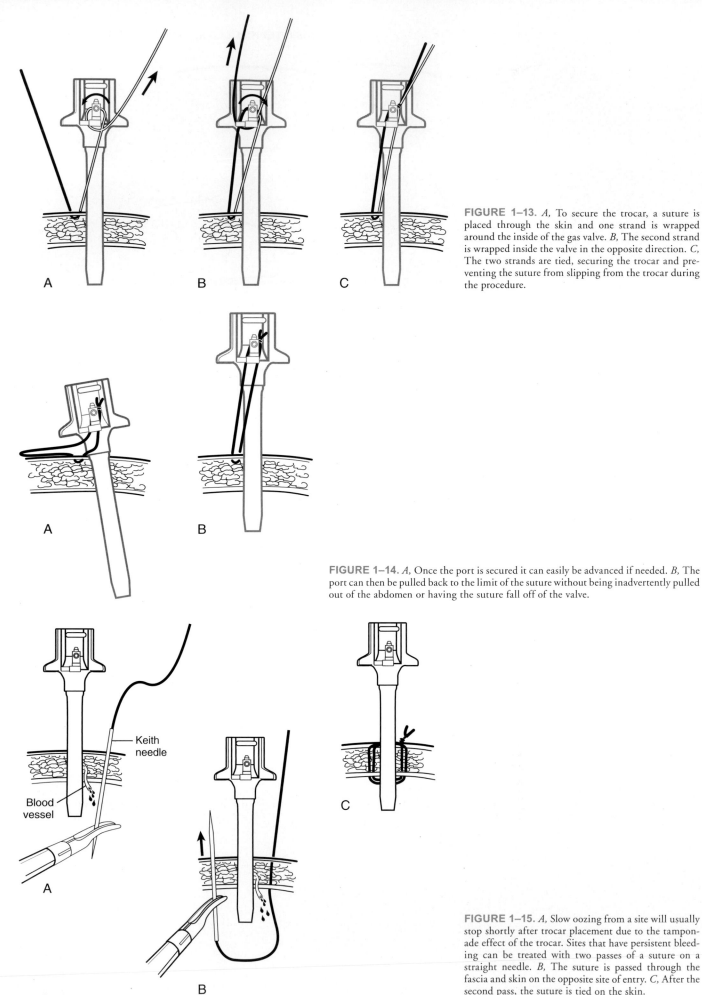

FIGURE 1–13. *A,* To secure the trocar, a suture is placed through the skin and one strand is wrapped around the inside of the gas valve. *B,* The second strand is wrapped inside the valve in the opposite direction. *C,* The two strands are tied, securing the trocar and preventing the suture from slipping from the trocar during the procedure.

FIGURE 1–14. *A,* Once the port is secured it can easily be advanced if needed. *B,* The port can then be pulled back to the limit of the suture without being inadvertently pulled out of the abdomen or having the suture fall off of the valve.

Keith needle

Blood vessel

FIGURE 1–15. *A,* Slow oozing from a site will usually stop shortly after trocar placement due to the tamponade effect of the trocar. Sites that have persistent bleeding can be treated with two passes of a suture on a straight needle. *B,* The suture is passed through the fascia and skin on the opposite site of entry. *C,* After the second pass, the suture is tied on the skin.

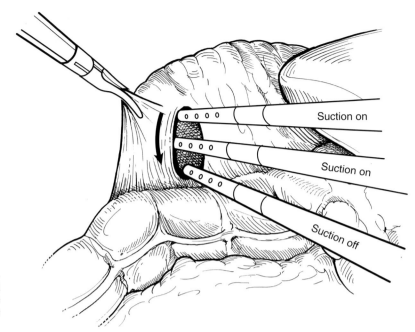

FIGURE 1–16. The irrigator aspirator is useful during dissection as a blunt instrument and aspirator. The tissue is trapped with the tip while suction is applied and then spread in the opposite direction of a second instrument. Once the tissue plane is opened, the suction is discontinued, releasing the tissue.

HEMOSTASIS

Electrocautery

Electrocautery was initially the mainstay for hemostasis during laparoscopic dissection, but it is slowly being replaced by other technologies. Nevertheless, an important role remains for electrocautery's safe use in laparoscopic surgery. Excessive bleeding from even small venous vessels can quickly obscure the surgical field, causing difficulty in finding correct planes of dissection. Surgery on retroperitoneal structures requires operating very close to bowel segments. In the retroperitoneal approach, bowel is not readily identified, but it is also in the area of dissection and subject to thermal injury. More than half of laparoscopic bowel injuries reported in the literature result from electrocautery insult. Thermal injury can be prevented by vigilant surveillance of contact points during dissection.[6]

Monopolar electrosurgery is the modality still commonly used in surgery. In the monopolar circuit, the active electrode is in the surgical site and the return electrode is the grounding pad. Consequently, the current passes through the body of the patient to complete the circuit (Fig. 1–17). The waveform can be continuous or intermittent (cut or coagulation) and is low current with high voltage. Avoid applying monopolar electricity to ductlike strands of tissue attached to bowel. A rise in temperature from electrocautery on these small bands from a short burst of energy can result is tissue death at the bowel segment.[7] Unrecognized bowel injuries can also occur because of stray energy released from breaks in the integrity of the insulated coating or capacitive coupling along the shaft of the instrument or trocar. These injuries can occur outside the surgeon's field of view[8] (Fig. 1–18).

The use of monopolar instruments and active electrode monitoring devices minimizes the chance of unrecognized thermal injury from insulation failure, direct coupling, and capacitive coupling. When an active electrode monitoring system (AEM active electrode monitoring system; Encision, Boulder, CO) detects stray energy, the electrosurgical generator is deactivated before injury can occur.

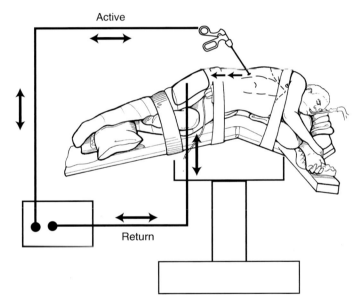

FIGURE 1–17. In a monopolar circuit the active electrode is in the surgical site and the return electrode is the grounding pad on the patient's skin. The current passes through the body of the patient to complete the circuit.

In bipolar electrosurgery, the active electrode and the return electrode functions are performed at the site of surgery between the tips of the instrument. The waveform is continuous, low current, and low voltage. Only the tissue grasped is included in the electrical circuit. The risk of injury from stray surgical energy is minimized with this system (Fig. 1–19).

Argon beam coagulation uses the properties of electrosurgery and a stream of argon gas to improve the effectiveness of the electrosurgical current. Argon gas is noncombustible and inert, making it a safe gas to use in the presence of electrosurgical current. The argon gas is ionized by the electrical current, making it more conductive than air. The highly conductive

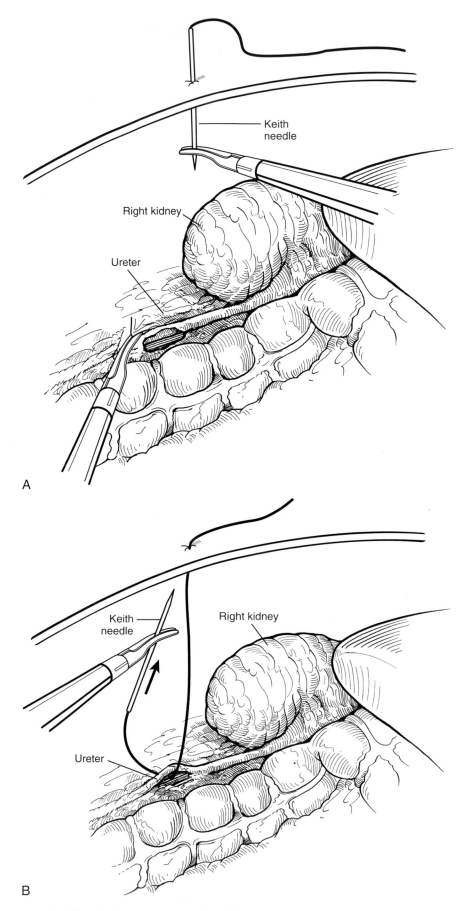

FIGURE 1–26. *A,* Retraction can be achieved without the insertion of an additional trocar site. When temporary retraction is needed, a straight needle with suture can be passed through the abdominal wall under direct vision. *B,* The needle is passed through or under the structure to be retracted.

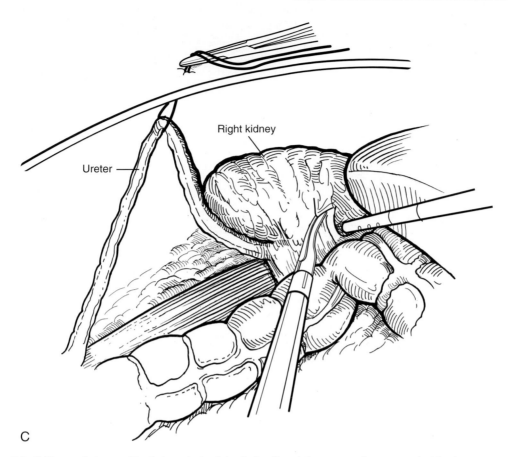

C

FIGURE 1–26, cont'd. *C*, The needle is passed back through the abdominal wall, and the two strands are secured with a hemostat.

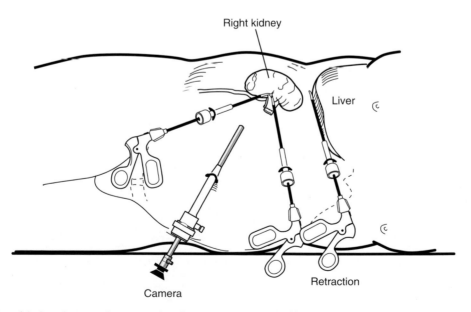

FIGURE 1–27. Retraction of the liver during nephrectomy, adrenalectomy, or retroperitoneal lymph node dissection can be accomplished through an additional 5-mm or 3-mm port placed in the midline below the xiphoid process or below the costal margin in the midclavicular line. Preferably, a locking grasper is available to pass under the liver and, after grasping the peritoneal edge on the right lateral side wall, can be locked in place, retracting the liver from the field of dissection.

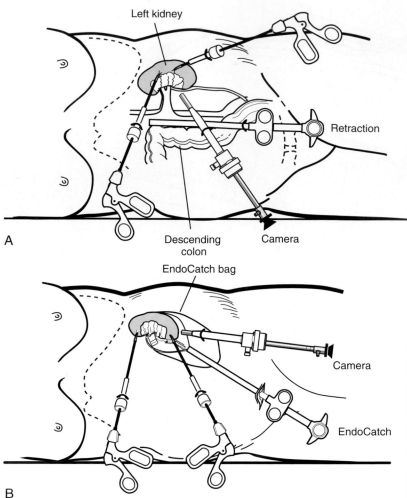

A

B

FIGURE 1–28. *A,* During a left-sided dissection where tissue is to be removed, a 10-mm or 15-mm EndoCatch II (U.S. Surgical, Norwalk, CT) can be inserted for assistance. For nephrectomy specimens, a 15-mm device is placed after a small incision has been created in the skin approximately two fingerbreadths above the symphysis pubis. A 10-mm trocar is then inserted to create the fascial tract and then removed. The 15-mm EndoCatch II, without a trocar, is then placed through the dilated site and used for retraction. The size difference between the trocar and the EndoCatch allows a snug fit against the skin that will prevent gas escape during the procedure. *B,* Once the kidney is freed, the bag is deployed, and the organ is entrapped and removed through a Pfannenstiel incision.

TABLE 1–1.   CHARACTERISTICS OF COMMERCIALLY AVAILABLE DEVICES FOR HAND-ASSISTED LAPAROSCOPY

Characteristic	GelPort	Lap Disc	Omniport
Manufacturer	Applied Medical, Rancho Santa Margarita, CA	Ethicon Endo-Surgery, Cincinnati, OH	Advanced Surgical Concepts, Ireland, distributed in United States by Weck Closure, Raleigh, NC
Device diameter	13 cm	12 cm	12 cm
Number of different sizes	2	2	1
Number of components	3 Pieces: Flexible skirt, rigid base, gel cap	1 Piece	2 Pieces: Cuff with retention rings, insufflation device
Advantages	Gel cap maintains pneumoperitoneum with or with out instruments and allows instrument to be placed directly though cap device	Small and simple to work. An iris configuration allows opening to be large enough for hand or tightly placed around a trocar	Able to maintain pneumoperitoneum even when incision is too long
Disadvantages	Gas leak if incision is too long	Gas leak if incision is too long	Loss of pneumoperitoneum when hand is removed
Cost per device	$575	$490	$415

From Wolf JS: Tips and tricks for hand-assisted surgery. AUA Update series 24:2, 2005; Rane A, Dasgupta P: Prospective experience with a second-generation hand-assisted laparoscopic device and comparison with first-generation devices. J Endourol 17:895–897, 2003; and Rupa P, Stifelman MD: Hand-assisted laparoscopic devices: The second generation. J Endourol 18:649–653, 2004.

instruments. The hand-assist devices offer a bridge between laparoscopic and open surgery and may offer assistance for surgeons without advanced laparoscopic training who still want to offer laparoscopic advantages with a small midline incision. Hand-assisted dissection may also be helpful in patients whose pathologic condition makes laparoscopy more difficult, such as infectious processes or prior surgery.

Sections on hand-assisted procedures are included in this atlas with specific details on placement and dissection outlined for each procedure.

RETRIEVAL

Anyone who has struggled to place an organ or tissue in a bag will immediately appreciate advances in retrieval technology.

The EndoCatch II is a self-opening bag that comes in several sizes including 10 mm and 15 mm. Once the instrument is placed through a trocar or directly through the skin, the inner core handle slides forward, advancing the bag. A metal band automatically opens the bag and can be used to scoop up the tissue to be removed. By pulling a separate string, the bag closes and tears away from the metal ring. The ring is pulled back into the handle and the device is removed, leaving the closed bag and string in the working space. The current bags are not strong enough to withstand automated tissue morcellation (Fig. 1–29).

The LapSac (Cook Urological, Spencer, IN) provides a sturdy nylon sac that allows the specimen to be morcellated with hand instruments. Placement of the organ into the LapSac is greatly facilitated by feeding a standard hydrophilic wire through the holes in the opening of the sac before inserting the

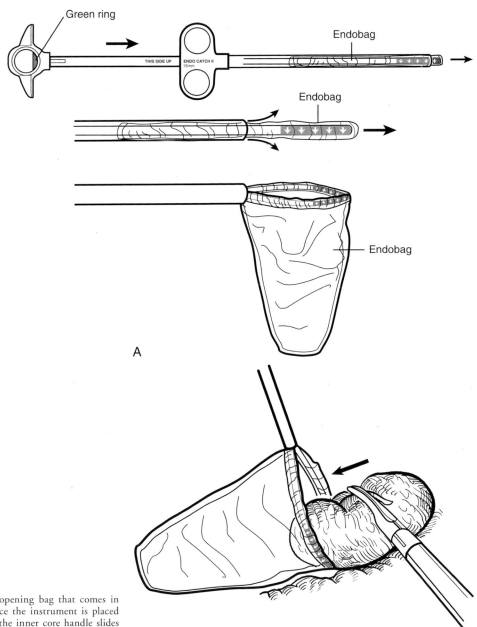

FIGURE 1–29. *A,* The EndoCatch is a self-opening bag that comes in several sizes including 10 mm and 15 mm. Once the instrument is placed through a trocar or directly through the skin, the inner core handle slides forward, advancing the bag. *B,* A metal band automatically springs the bag open and can be used to scoop up the tissue to be removed.

Continued

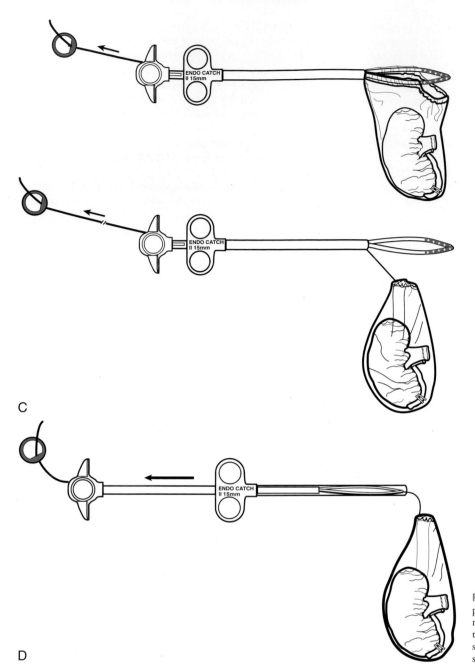

C

D

FIGURE 1–29, cont'd. *C,* A separate string is pulled, closing the bag and tearing it away from the metal ring. *D,* The metal ring is retracted back inside the sleeve, leaving the bag and string behind. The string is cut, leaving a long strand exiting the trocar site.

sac into the abdomen. Roll the sac and place it through the skin into the abdomen through a 12-mm trocar site with the trocar removed. The ends of the wire remain outside the abdomen. Then place the trocar back through the 12-mm skin incision. Using two instruments, unroll and open the sac, and use the wire to help hold the mouth open. After moving the specimen inside the sac, withdraw the wire and close the opening with the LapSac string. Then pull the sac through a 12-mm trocar site; I usually enlarge the site to approximately 2 cm. As the sac is pulled open, the entrapped tissue is seen at the opening. Using alternating bites with a ring forceps and Kocher clamp, carefully morcellate the tissue. Only grasp tissue crowning at the opening. Do not make deep passes into the LapSac because bowel outside of the sac can be inadvertently grasped and damaged.

For lymph node dissection and other procedures in which tissue is going to be extracted, a 10-mm EndoCatch can be used in a similar fashion without a trocar or passed through a 10-mm port inserted 2 fingerbreadths above the symphysis pubis. In addition, a 15-mm EndoCatch can be placed through a 15-mm Thoracoport (U.S. Surgical, Norwalk, CT) to maintain pneumoperitoneum during the procedure.

MECHANICAL ASSISTANCE

The Automated Endoscopic System for Optimal Positioning, or AESOP, robotic device (Computer Motion Inc., Goleta, CA) is a voice-activated assistant that holds and positions the camera for the surgeon during the procedure. The robot provides a

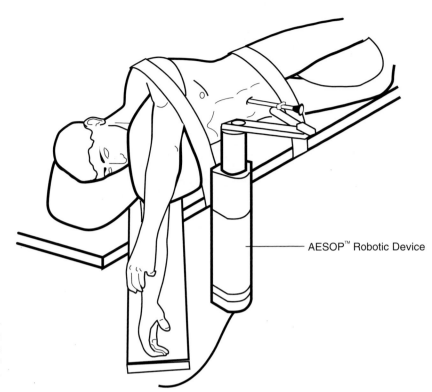

AESOP™ Robotic Device

FIGURE 1–30. The AESOP Robotic Device (Computer Motion Inc., Goleta, CA) is a voice-activated assistant that holds and positions the camera for the surgeon during the procedure. The robot provides a motionless image, and the field of view is changed at the surgeon's command through use of a headset and the voice recognition system.

motionless image and the field of view is changed at the surgeon's command through a headset and the voice recognition system (Fig. 1–30).

The TISKA (Trocar and Instrument Positioning System) Endoarm (TISKA Endoarm; Karl Storz, Endoskope, Tuttlingen, Germany) is a system developed to assist with trocar and instrument positioning. This device maintains the position of the trocar sheath at a fixed point at the trocar puncture site while instruments or laparoscopes are changed or removed. Routine laparoscopic needs such as tissue retraction can easily be performed with this system. The TISKA Endoarm is not currently available in the United States.

INTRAOPERATIVE IMAGING

New advances in ultrasound technology allow laparoscopic imaging in many different situations. Intraoperative laparoscopic ultrasonography allows the surgeon to determine the presence of multifocal renal lesions or to evaluate complex cystic masses (Fig. 1–31). The presence of a renal vein tumor thrombus can be readily detected during nephrectomy, and appropriate measures must be taken to ensure adequate treatment. In some adrenalectomy cases and renal biopsy cases in the morbidly obese, the organ can be difficult to locate without intraoperative imaging.

New generations of laparoscopic US probes also allow needle biopsy of suspicious lesions through the probe (B-K Medical, Herlev, Denmark) (Fig. 1–32).

RETROPERITONEAL ACCESS

A transabdominal approach to retroperitoneal structures is preferred in most procedures. The transperitoneal approach is more familiar for the surgeon and allows immediate visualization of important anatomic landmarks.

Adipose tissue in the retroperitoneum and a small working space can be considerable visual barriers to rapid progress of the surgical procedure. In a transabdominal approach, the anatomic planes of dissection are similar to open surgery, making this approach easier for the beginning laparoscopic surgeon and resident-in-training to overcome the learning curve associated with this new skill.

Nevertheless, there are patients in whom retroperitoneal access is preferred. The patient with a history of multiple abdominal surgical procedures, in whom mesh for abdominal wall closure has been used, or with a history of peritonitis may benefit from this approach. The patient with a posterior exophytic cyst or mass may be better served through retroperitoneal access. Consequently, the laparoscopic surgeon needs to be familiar with both transperitoneal and retroperitoneal access.

There are several different methods to gain retroperitoneal access. Place the patient in the lateral decubitus position with the table flexed and the kidney rest extended; this increases the distance between the 12th rib and the anterior superior iliac crest. At the tip of the 12th rib, make a 1.5- to 2-cm incision and spread it down to the lumbodorsal fascia. Also incise the fascia and extend your index finger to create a working space toward the kidney or adrenal gland. Insert a handmade or commercial balloon system into the space and direct it toward the area of dissection. Instill normal saline in the balloon to create a 500- to 800-mL working space. After several minutes, deflate the balloon, insert a 10-mm Hasson trocar, and create the pneumoretroperitoneum (Fig. 1–33).

Instead of the balloon and Hasson trocar method, a trocar with a visual obturator can be used to access the retroperitoneum through a standard 1-cm incision. Once the trocar is in place and connected to the insufflator, insert the camera through the trocar and use it to bluntly push the peritoneum

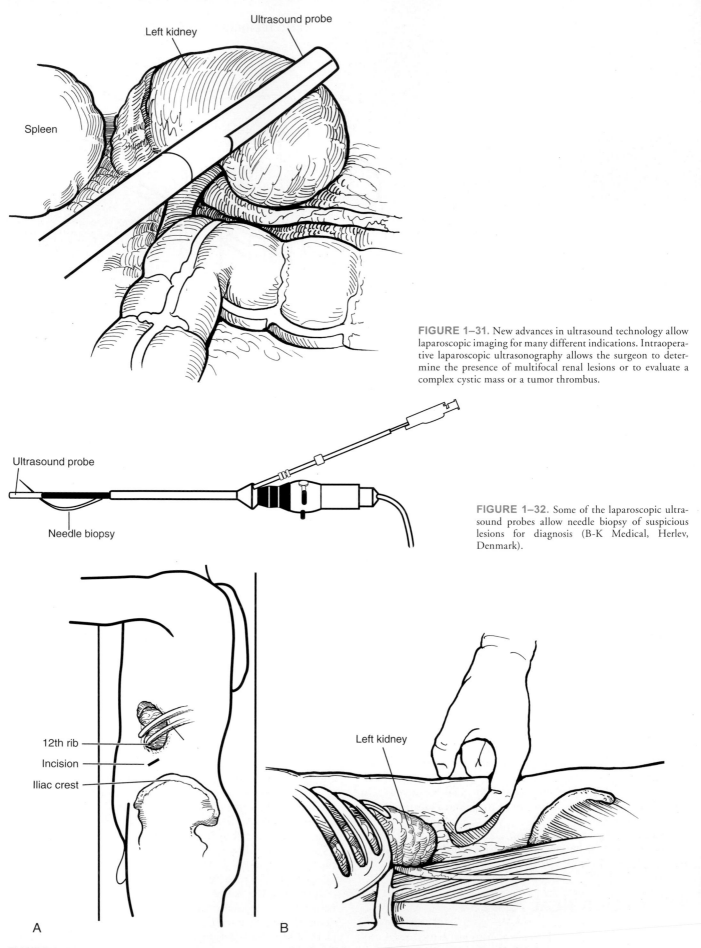

FIGURE 1–31. New advances in ultrasound technology allow laparoscopic imaging for many different indications. Intraoperative laparoscopic ultrasonography allows the surgeon to determine the presence of multifocal renal lesions or to evaluate a complex cystic mass or a tumor thrombus.

FIGURE 1–32. Some of the laparoscopic ultrasound probes allow needle biopsy of suspicious lesions for diagnosis (B-K Medical, Herlev, Denmark).

FIGURE 1–33. *A,* To gain retroperitoneal access, the patient is placed in the lateral decubitis position with the table flexed and the kidney rest extended. This increases the distance between the 12th rib and the anterior superior iliac crest. At the tip of the 12th rib, a 1.5- to 2-cm incision is created and spread down to the lumbodorsal fascia. *B,* The fascia is also incised, and the surgeon's index finger is extended to create a working space toward the kidney or adrenal gland.

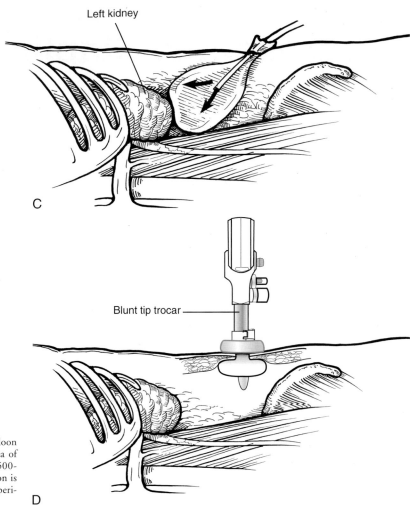

FIGURE 1–33, cont'd. *C,* A handmade or commercial balloon system is inserted into the space and directed toward the area of dissection. Normal saline is instilled in the balloon to create a 500- to 800-mL working space. *D,* After several minutes, the balloon is deflated, a 10-mm Hasson trocar is inserted, and pneumoretroperitoneum is created.

medially. The expanding working space is maintained by CO_2 as the scope is used to open tissue planes under direct vision.

Insert additional trocars according to the particular procedure being performed. Descriptions of the retroperitoneal approach (in addition to the transabdominal approach) are included in subsequent chapters on adrenalectomy, renal biopsy, and renal cyst decortication.

SUMMARY

Techniques in laparoscopic surgery have changed rapidly over the past 15 years, due in large part to advances in equipment. New technologies for trocar insertion, dissection, hemostasis, retraction, tissue retrieval, suturing, stapling, and intraoperative imaging have improved the ability to perform more complex laparoscopic surgeries.

REFERENCES

1. Graff TD, Arbegast NR, Phillips OC, et al: Gas embolism: A comparative study of air and carbon dioxide as embolic agents in the systemic venous system. Am J Obstet Gynecol 78:259–265, 1959.
2. Wolf SJ, Marshall LS: The physiology of laparoscopy: Basic principles, complications, and other considerations. J Urol 152:294, 1994.
3. Wittgen CM, Andrus CH, Fitzgerald SD, et al: Analysis of the hemodynamic and ventilatory effects of laparoscopic cholecystectomy. Arch Surg 126:997–1001, 1991.
4. Wehlage MB: Anesthetic implications of laparoscopy, thoracoscopy and hysteroscopy. In Arregui ME, Fitzgibbons RJ Jr (eds): Principles of Laparoscopic Surgery: Basic and Advanced Techniques. New York, Springer-Verlag, 1995, pp 79–86.
5. Shekarriz H, Shekarriz B, Upadhyay J, et al: Experimental laparoscopic partial nephrectomy: Hydro-jet dissection: A porcine model initial experience. J Urol 161:4S, 1999.
6. Bishoff JT, Allaf ME, Kirkels W, et al: Laparoscopic bowel injury: Incidence and clinical presentation. J Urol 161:887, 1999.
7. Saye WB, Miller W, Hertzman P: Electrosurgery thermal injury: Myth or misconception? Surg Laparosc Endosc 4:223, 1991.
8. Grosskinsky CM, Hulka JE: Unipolar electrosurgery in operative laparoscopy. Capacitance as a potential source of injury. J Reprod Med 40:549, 1995.
9. Nakada S, Moon T, Gist M, et al: Use of the pneumosleeve as an adjunct in laparoscopic nephrectomy. Urology 49:612–613, 1997.
10. Wolf JS, Marcovich R, Gill IS, et al: Survey of neuromuscular injuries to the patient and surgeon during urologic laparoscopic surgery. Urology 55:831, 2000.
11. Batker R, Schoor R, Gonzalez C, et al: Hand-assisted laparoscopic radical nephrectomy: The experience of the inexperienced. J Endourol 15:513–516, 2001.
12. Wolf JS: Tips and tricks for hand-assisted surgery. AUA Update Series 24:2, 2005.
13. Rane A, Dasgupta P: Prospective experience with a second-generation hand-assisted laparoscopic device and comparison with first-generation devices. J Endourol 17:895–897, 2003.

CHAPTER 2

Laparoscopic Stapling and Reconstruction

Gyan Pareek
Stephen Y. Nakada

Since the introduction of the laparoscopic nephrectomy in 1991 by Clayman and colleagues,[1] urologists have accepted that extirpative laparoscopic renal surgery is the first-line approach in most cases. Recent advancements in equipment technology have increased the laparoscopic applications in urology to more reconstructive type of procedures, including ureterolysis, ureteroureterostomy, nephropexy, pyeloplasty, and radical prostatectomy.

As with any type of surgery, methods and devices for hemostasis and tissue approximation are vital in laparoscopic surgery. Laparoscopic stapling and clipping devices are available for ligating vessels, approximating peritoneum, placing mesh, closing a viscus, and obliterating a lumen. Like their open-surgery counterparts, these devices were developed as faster, more efficient alternatives to hand suturing. Because intracorporeal suturing and knot tying are essential to nearly all these procedures, mastering these skills is essential for the retroperitoneal surgeon. This chapter provides a detailed description of the various clips, staples, and suturing techniques required to perform these laparoscopic urologic procedures.

CLIPS

Equipment

Occlusive clips are ideal for smaller arteries and veins and are now standard equipment in all laparoscopic procedures. As in open surgery, clips provide a rapid alternative for hemostasis. Today, most endoscopic clips are titanium, and they vary in size from 5 to 12 mm. There are absorbable clips, and some research shows no difference in adhesion formation between metallic and absorbable clips.[2]

The actual clips have characteristic ridges and valleys stamped onto the surface that is in contact with the tissue. Ideally, the variegated pattern prevents the clip from being dislodged by increased vascular pressure or by subsequent nearby tissue dissection. An occlusive clip starts out in a V shape; as it is squeezed by the applier, the tips close first, from distal to proximal (Fig. 2–1). This manner of closing ensures that the entire structure to be ligated is contained within the clip. Nonabsorbable polymer ligating clips (Weck Closure Systems, Research Triangle Park, NC) are also available (Fig. 2–2). These clips perform the same function as sutures by penetrating and locking through multiple layers of tissue. The engaging clip latching mechanism allows the surgeon to feel and hear the clip close. Use of the polymer ligating clip has been reported to be safe for renal artery ligation during nephrectomy.[3]

Occlusive clip appliers can be broadly classified into various categories: multiple load or single load and disposable or multiple use. Originally, the standard clip applier was single load and multiple use. The main advantage of the reusable units is their cost savings after initial investment. The disadvantages of these older models follow:

1. Extra time to exit and reenter the abdomen to load the clips
2. Tendency for loaded clips to fall from the jaws as they pass through the trocar
3. Lack of rotating shafts
4. Initial cost, which is four to six times that of disposable units

AutoSuture (U.S. Surgical, Norwalk, CT) offers a multiple-load, multiple-use model. However, this device is not as widely used because the multiple-load tools do not withstand the rigors of stocking, resterilization, and multiple uses.

The majority of laparoscopic clip appliers used today are single use and multiple load, carrying between 15 and 30 clips per unit (Table 2–1). The ability to fire multiple clips without exiting the abdomen to reload can save significant time and minimize blood loss in the case of clipping a bleeding vessel.

The diameter of the shaft generally depends on the size of the clips. Shafts of 5 mm are available for medium clip appliers. The EndoClip 5-mm shaft, single-use clip applier (Ethicon Endo-Surgery, Cincinnati, OH) can deliver a slightly larger clip than other 5-mm clippers; its hinged jaws are normally retracted within the shaft, but when the handles are squeezed, the jaws advance and expand and a clip is automatically loaded. Otherwise, for medium-large and large clips, the shaft sizes are 10 mm and 12 mm, respectively.

In addition to their multiple-load capabilities, the disposable units have several other notable features. First, 360-degree rotating shafts are present on nearly all appliers. This important feature allows the handle of the instrument to lie comfortably in the hand while the applier's tips are placed around the target tissue at an ideal angle. No articulating clip appliers are currently available. Second, automatically loading clips, which are available in many models, eliminate another step in clip application; immediately after a clip is placed, another one is advanced into firing position. Also, the automatically loading clips do not fall from the applier's jaws while being passed through the trocar as easily as from the single-load, multiple-use appliers. One potential disadvantage of automatic clip loading is that the tips of the clip applier cannot be used as a dissecting tool without possibly dislodging the unfired clip into the field. However, some clippers require the user to pull a trigger on the handle to load the clip. On newer models, the clip is loaded only when the surgeon begins to close the handles, without the requirement of pulling a separate lever. Third, most new models have a visual indicator to alert the user that only a few clips are left. A safety feature that is not available in all appliers is an automatic lock that prevents the jaws from closing when the device is out of clips.

Instrument Use

The vessel or other structure to be clipped is dissected until the entire structure can be contained within the clip without a significant amount of interceding tissue. This step prevents the clip from slipping off and ensures that it has maximal contact with and pressure on the vessel. Also, the dissected window must be large enough to allow placement of several clips, with enough room left over to divide the structure with endoscopic scissors. On a small- to medium-sized vessel, one or two clips on either side usually suffice. For larger structures (e.g., renal artery), three clips are applied proximally and two clips distally before the vessel is divided.

Before placing the jaws around the tissue, ensure that there is a clip in place because closing the jaws without a clip could sever the structure. Once the clip applier's jaws completely surround the structure and the tips are easily seen, gently squeeze the handle until the tips of the clip just meet (Fig. 2–3). Then slide the clip up or down the structure for ideal positioning and finish by firmly squeezing the handle.

Withdraw the clip applier at the same angle used for the approach to avoid accidentally pulling off the clip. The Ligaclip Allport 5-mm clip applier (Ethicon Endo-Surgery) has a hinged jaw and uses a unique clip (see Fig. 2–2). After applying the clip, a small lip on the tip of the serrated jaw (see Fig. 2–3)

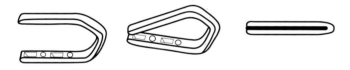

FIGURE 2–1. Standard laparoscopic clip closes from distal to proximal, with tips touching first.

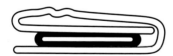

FIGURE 2–2. Hem-o-lok (Weck Closure Systems, Research Triangle Park, NC) nonabsorbable polymer ligating clip.

requires the user to back off the clip before withdrawing the applier to avoid dislodging the clip. If the clip is misplaced, use a Maryland-style forceps to withdraw it through the port.

Place additional clips as necessary, then use laparoscopic scissors to divide the tissue. Avoid using electrocautery to divide the vessels in order to avoid tissue necrosis and late failing of the clips. On larger vessels, we prefer to place clips in an alternating fashion so that the tips of the clips are facing opposite directions. A right-angle clip applier is ideal for this purpose and for other hard-to-reach structures. With current technology, the height of the clip and jaws limit the right-angle clip applier to 10-mm ports.

BITING CLIPS AND SINGLE STAPLES

Equipment

Use biting or tacking clips and staples to rapidly approximate tissue and to fix mesh without needing to place many individual sutures. Laparoscopic biting staplers originally were developed to repair laparoscopic hernia with mesh, but these devices are also useful in refashioning the peritoneum in laparoscopic ureterolysis and fixing mesenteric defects in bowel resections. Much like the staplers used for skin wound closure, laparoscopic staplers fire titanium staples with sharp ends that enter the tissue and then undergo deformation into either a **B** shape or a rectangle (Fig. 2–4).

Most contemporary devices are single-use and multiple-load, with 15 to 30 staples per unit. Disposable staplers typically cost more than those for the single-load reusable models, but the multiple-load feature makes their use much more efficient than withdrawing the instrument for each new biting clip to be placed. If the surgeon needs more than the 15 to 30 staples originally loaded, many new staplers allow for reloads, rather than requiring the use of another unit. A 360-degree rotating shaft is essential for accurate placement of the staple while allowing the squeeze-handle to rest comfortably in the hand. Some devices also come with a 60- to 65-degree distal articulating head, which permits the stapling of hard-to-reach areas like the anterior abdominal wall and deep pelvis.

Firing a Biting Clip: Technique

To reapproximate the peritoneum, as during intraperitonealization in a laparoscopic ureterolysis, introduce the biting stapler through its 10/12-mm port, which is ideally at a 90-degree angle with the target surface.

TABLE 2–1.   DISPOSABLE, MULTIPLE-LOAD SINGLE-USE LAPAROSCOPIC CLIP APPLIERS

	Ligaclip Allport	Ligaclip Right-Angle	Ligaclip MCA	EndoClip	EndoClip II	EndoClip Multapplier
Manufacturer	Ethicon Endo-Surgery	Ethicon Endo-Surgery	Ethicon Endo-Surgery	AutoSuture	AutoSuture	AutoSuture
Port size (mm)	5	10	12	5	10	10
No. of clips	20–30	20	20	20	20	8
Sizes of clip	Medium, medium-large, or large	Medium-large	Large	Medium-large	Medium-large, large	Medium-large, large
Clip loading	Automatic	Automatic	Automatic	Separate lever	Automatic	Automatic

Ethicon Endo-Surgery, Inc., Cincinnati, OH; AutoSuture, U.S. Surgical, Norwalk, CT.

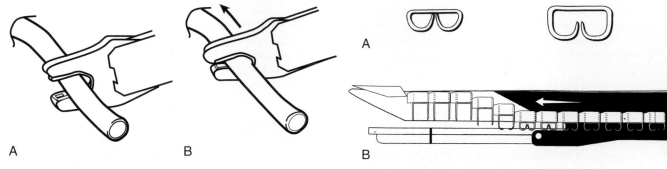

FIGURE 2–3. Clip ligation of a vessel. The jaws are closed until the tips meet *(A)* and then closed and moved proximally and closed tightly to occlude vessel *(B)*.

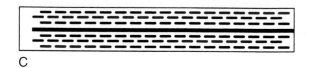

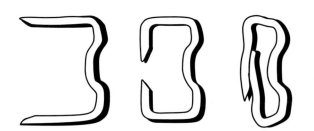

FIGURE 2–4. Biting clip deforms to a final rectangular shape.

FIGURE 2–5. Linear staplers. *A,* Vascular staple forms a tighter **B** shape than a regular or thick staple. *B,* Linear stapler jaws, side view: Upon firing of the stapler, staples are forced downwards against the anvil and conform to their characteristic shape. The staples continue past the cut line to ensure hemostasis. *C,* Standard load: Three parallel rows of staples on either side of the cut line.

Before grasping and reapproximating the peritoneum, position the stapling head at approximately the anticipated angle of stapling. This maneuver avoids prolonged traction on and tearing of the tissue. With an articulating stapler, angle the head so that the distal articulating shaft is perpendicular to the surface; then rotate the shaft until the firing head is at a right angle to the defect.

Next, secure each free peritoneal edge with separate graspers and pull the edges together until they meet. Poise the stapler head over the two edges and squeeze the handle gently only until five or six "clicks" are felt and the two staple tips protruding from the end of the stapler head can be seen.

Advance the points of the staple into the tissue and squeeze the handle the rest of the way. Once a few clips have been placed, only a single grasper may be needed to reapproximate the peritoneal edges.

LINEAR STAPLERS

Equipment

Laparoscopic linear staplers are vital tools for rapid, safe intracorporeal tissue division and reapproximation of visceral structures. With the squeeze of a handle, such a device deploys multiple, closely spaced, parallel rows of titanium staples.

Staples come in three different "loads"—thin/vascular, medium, and large/thick—and are color-coded for easy recognition.

1. *Thin/vascular* staples penetrate tissue to a depth of 2 to 2.5 mm, deform to an exaggerated B shape, and form a reli-

ably hemostatic staple line; they are ideal for rapidly ligating vascular pedicles and dividing thin, vascular mesentery.
2. *Medium* staples are 3.0 to 3.9 mm thick in their closed form and are useful in securing thicker tissues such as bowel, bladder, and ureter.
3. *Large* staples are 4.0 to 4.8 mm thick in their closed form and are also useful in securing thicker tissues. Larger staples do not fold to the same tight shape as small staples, and are not used for primarily hemostatic ligation.

Staples find their final shape as follows. With the target tissue secured between the two jaws of the stapler, staples are forced out of the load, through the tissue, and against an opposing anvil, where they reflect back upon themselves (Fig. 2–5).

Several years ago, a stapler could be reloaded only four times before its inner workings became unreliable (or the knife too dull) and it had to be discarded. Staplers today allow the same instrument to fire between 8 and 25 separate loads before disposal (Table 2–2).

Linear staplers can be broadly classified into cutting and noncutting staplers. *Cutting* versions deploy loads with six intercalated parallel rows of staples. As the staples are fired, a knife follows closely behind and incises the tissue down the middle of the load, leaving three rows of staples on each side. The staple line extends past the range of the cutting knife by one or two staples to avoid incising nonsecured tissue (see Fig. 2–5). Once the staples are fired, a safety feature on all such devices prevents accidental redeployment of the cutting knife until a new load with staples is in place. *Noncutting* staplers, which simply fire three or four parallel rows of staples, are useful for closing enterotomies and repairing bladder injuries.

Laparoscopic linear cutting staplers are further distinguished by the length of their staple line (30/35, 45, and 60 mm) and whether or not their firing heads are articulated. An articulating head gives a greater range of motion from a fixed trocar

TABLE 2–2. LINEAR STAPLERS

	Endopath ETS	Endopath ETS-Flex Articulating	Endopath EZ45: Cutter	Endopath EZ45: No-Knife	Multifire Endo GIA 30	Multifire Endo TA 30	Endo GIA Universal
Manufacturer	Ethicon Endo-Surgery	Ethicon Endo-Surgery	Ethicon Endo-Surgery	Ethicon Endo-Surgery	U.S. Surgical	U.S. Surgical	
Port size (mm)	12	12	12	12	12	12	12
Staple size(s)	Vascular/thin, regular	Vascular/thin, regular	Regular, thick	Regular, thick	2.0, 2.5, and 3.5 mm	2.5 and 3.5 mm	2.0, 2.5, 3.5, and 4.8 mm
Staple length(s) (mm)	35	35	45	45	30	30	30, 45, and 60
Rotating shaft	Yes	Yes	Yes	Yes	Yes	Yes	Yes
Articulating	No	Yes	No	No	No	No	Yes

Ethicon Endo-Surgery, Inc., Cincinnati, OH; U.S. Surgical, Norwalk, CT.

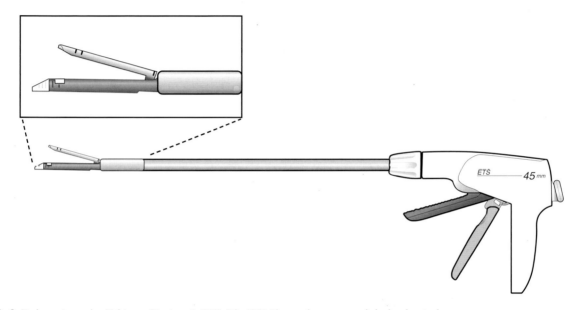

FIGURE 2–6. Endoscopic stapler (Ethicon, Cincinnati, OH). The ETS-Flex stapler rotates and the head articulates.

but adds to the stapler's price. All devices offer a rotating shaft, which is essential for proper visualization of the tips during firing.

On most models, a replacement load consists of a fresh six rows of staples but uses the same knife and anvil inherent to the actual stapling device. The ETS-Flex stapler (Ethicon, Cincinnati, OH) is illustrated in Figure 2–6. The stapler is unique in that the head of the stapler articulates, allowing application at various angles.

The minimum size limitation imposed by the width of the staple load requires use of a 10-mm or larger port for all currently available staplers.

Firing a Linear Stapler: Technique

Choose the appropriate stapler or staple load according to the following criteria:

1. Accessibility of the tissue to be stapled
2. Tissue thickness
3. Whether the tissue is vascular or nonvascular
4. Whether a cutting or noncutting staple is needed

Introduce the stapler with its jaws closed through a 12- or 15-mm port under direct vision and then observe through the laparoscope while moving the stapler to the prepared site. Ideally, watch the stapler head from the side; do not look down the shaft of the instrument. Then rotate the shaft and use any articulating features to position the head of the stapler. The jaw holding the staple load is on the back of the instrument, ready to be passed through the tissue window once the jaws are opened.

Next, retract the target tissue with graspers to open the tissue window, open the jaws of the stapler, and pass the jaw holding the staple load through the window. The end of most staplers can be used to perform some additional blunt dissection as necessary. Advance the jaws of the stapler until the tips are well beyond the far edge of the tissue and close the jaws to their locked position. If too much tissue is included, the jaws may not be parallel after being closed. This situation poses a risk that the distal staples will not come in contact with the anvil and thus will not conform to the appropriate B shape. With the stapler's jaws locked, observe that the so-called cut lines printed on either side of the stapler's head are distal to the tissue to be incised. There are safety measures built into each model that must be deployed before firing the staples.

Next, fire the staples, reopen the jaws before withdrawing the instrument from the staple site, and immediately ensure that the staple line is intact and occlusive. Finally, close the handles under direct vision with the laparoscope and remove the instrument for another load if necessary. The proper use of the stapler is essential because malfunction can lead to devastating consequences. Chan and associates[4] reported a 1.7% stapler malfunction rate (10 of 565 cases) during laparoscopic nephrectomies performed over a 10-year period. Interestingly, 7 of the 10 malfunctions may have been attributed to misuse of the stapling device.

LOOP LIGATION

Equipment and Use

Loop ligatures are most valuable in securing an already transected pedicle. Pass a length of suture with a preformed sliding, locking knot intracorporeally, whether self-tied or commercially prepared. Then retract the structure to be ligated through the loop with a grasper, and cinch the loop down with a knot pusher (Fig. 2–7).

Any slipknot can be used, but it must be reliable and must not backslide once cinched tight. One popular knot is the Roeder knot (Fig. 2–8), which was first used for loop ligation in tonsillectomy. A reliable knot, it can be made even stronger by throwing an extra half-hitch after tying the main body of the knot. Use a sliding knot pusher to advance the knot. Once the loop is in place around the tissue, pull back the free proximal end of the suture through the pusher to cinch the knot. To ensure the tightest knot possible, keep the tip of the pusher in tight apposition to the tissue while closing the loop. Depending on the size of the knot pusher and trocar, a reducing sleeve is often required to prevent leaking from the trocar site when the knot pusher is advanced into the body.

Two popular prefabricated loop ligature systems are Surgitie (U.S. Surgical, Norwalk, CT) and EndoLoop (Ethicon Endo-Surgery, Somerville, NJ). The Surgitie kit contains a reducing sleeve for a 5-mm port, a knot pusher, and a preloaded suture with loop. Pass the knot pusher and attached loop through the reducing shaft and then through the trocar, and advance them to the surgical site. Next, an assistant passes a grasper through the loop, locks its jaws on the tissue to be ligated, and retracts

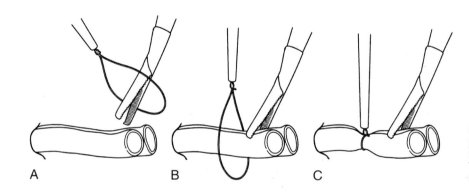

A   B   C

FIGURE 2–7. Loop ligation is performed with (*A*) a preformed loop that is passed into the body. *B*, The tissue to be ligated is grasped and pulled through the loop. *C*, The knot is cinched tight with a knot pusher three or four times.

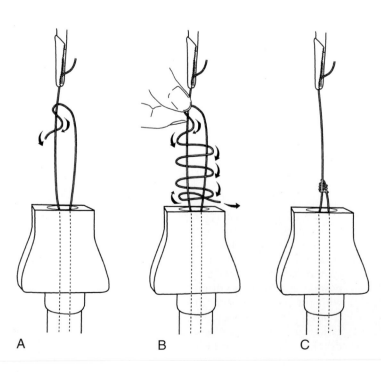

A   B   C

FIGURE 2–8. The Roeder knot is a sliding, locking knot used to create a preformed loop and for extracorporeal knot tying. *A*, Simple half-stitch is thrown. *B*, Half-stitch is pinched between the thumb and the forefinger, and the free end of the suture is passed around the two strands three to seven times. The free end of the suture is passed through the two strands and the knot is tightened. *C*, Finished knot with the free end trimmed.

the tissue back through the loop. (Alternatively, if the tissue is not retractile, the loop may be advanced distally along the length of the grasper's shaft.) With the knot ready to be cinched, snap off the proximal 2 cm of the plastic knot pusher, breaking the shaft into two pieces. With one hand, pull back the short proximal piece with attached suture while using the other hand to advance the knot pusher over the suture. Finally, cinch the knot two or three times and cut the suture.

The advantage of this prefabricated loop ligature system is that it requires no setup and is ready to use right out of the package. Available suture materials are both 0 and 2-0 plain gut, chromic gut, polyester, and synthetic absorbable varieties. The plastic knot pusher is available in only one length and may be too short to reach the target site if the wrong port is chosen. One minor inconvenience of this and other similar systems is that both hands are needed to cinch the knot, thus requiring an assistant to grasp the tissue and hold it still.

The EndoLoop loop ligature device is part of a larger endoscopic suturing system called EndoSuture (Ethicon Endo-Surgery). Unlike the disposable knot pusher and reducing sheath in other systems, the reusable metal EndoHandle and associated metal shaft can be reloaded with a variety of different sutures: EndoLoop ligature, needle with preformed loop, or simple suture-needle combination (Fig. 2–9A and B). With the EndoLoop suture loaded, pass the EndoHandle shaft through a 5-mm trocar, and introduce the loop to the surgical site. Once the loop is around the tissue and ready to be tightened, pull the proximal end of the suture backward. At the same time, the EndoHandle shaft with its disposable tapered plastic tip pushes the knot into the tissue and closes the loop. The proximal end of the suture is attached to a plastic button that is designed to be slid along the EndoSuture handle using only the thumb. This one-handed loop-tightening feature leaves one hand free for other tasks, such as grasping and retracting. Other advantages of this system are the reusable handle, generous shaft length, and 5-mm trocar compatibility without the need for a reducing sheath. This system has two minor drawbacks: (1) the extra time it takes to load the suture onto the EndoHandle and (2) the tendency to cause CO_2 leakage from the rubber trocar seal.

Although commercially preformed loops cost more than a length of suture, they save precious operating room minutes and are the preferred means of loop ligation.

LAPAROSCOPIC SUTURING

The introduction of occlusive clips, linear staples, tacking clips, and preformed loops has greatly aided laparoscopic surgery. Despite this technology, the laparoscopic surgeon must be able to efficiently perform simple-interrupted and running suture closures. The special limitations in laparoscopic surgery make this task among the most difficult to master, including fixed port sites, limited field of view (especially with new 5-mm–port scopes), two-dimensional monitor image under the control of another operator, and difficulty maintaining a bloodless field.

The ideal laparoscopic suturing device allows the surgeon to place a stitch at any angle despite trocar position and then automatically throw a perfect, reliable knot. This product does not exist, but several available devices make the task easier. Each device is discussed in the context of performing a simple-interrupted stitch and running suture line.

Preparation for Suturing

A minimum of three ports (preferably four) are needed for laparoscopic suturing: two ports for the needle driver and assisting grasper, one for the laparoscope and camera, and one for retracting tissue or suctioning. Choose the needle driver port so that the shaft of the driver is nearly parallel with the length of the wound. Locate the assisting grasper port at least 10 cm from the needle driver port to prevent the so-called crossing-swords phenomenon. Finally, place the laparoscope port so that the left-handed and right-handed instruments move the same way on the video image as they do in real life.

Ideally, these requirements involve placing the camera port between the two working ports. However, this placement often makes it difficult for the assistant (who is often on the other side of the table) to control the camera and perform retraction at the same time. The alternative is to place the camera port lateral to the two working ports. Avoid placing the camera port so that it is looking back on the working instruments; this arrangement makes suturing very difficult because the left- and right-hand movements are reversed on the monitor.

Take advantage of the laparoscope's magnification ability by using close-up views when actually placing the sutures. Moving the camera closer to the surgical site reduces the depth of field, thus minimizing the constraints of a two-dimensional image.

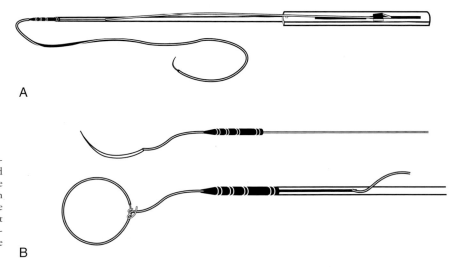

FIGURE 2–9. EndoSuture system (Ethicon, Cincinnati, OH). *A,* Metal handle and shaft with needle and suture load. A plastic knob at the proximal end of the suture fits into the groove on the handle. This knob can be slid up the handle with the surgeon's thumb to take up slack while the shaft is advanced during knot advancement. *B,* Close-up of the shaft tip with the preformed loop created by sliding the plastic knob on the handle.

Wide-angle shots are good for intracorporeal suture tying and for picking up the needle.

Sutures and Needles

Choice of suture in laparoscopy depends on the thickness and texture of tissue and whether sutures are to be permanent or absorbable. These considerations are similar to those in open procedures. For freehand suturing techniques, nearly all types of suture and needles are available. Choices are more limited for the use of the newer suturing devices.

As with open surgery, make more knots with monofilament sutures to avoid slipping. Handle suture carefully with atraumatic graspers to avoid fraying braided sutures and kinking monofilaments. Take extra care with the suture because the suture is handled by more instruments during laparoscopic surgery.

The length of suture for a particular knot or type of suture is another important consideration. For extracorporeal knotting, the suture is between 60 and 120 cm long to allow for passage through the trocar to the surgical site and back out through the same trocar. Shorter lengths are used for intracorporeal knotting to speed knot tying and minimize the amount of suture pulled through tissue. For a simple stitch, the suture length is 10 to 15 cm, with 12 mm added for each additional stitch in a running suture.

Laparoscopic needles come in different shapes: straight, curved, ski-shaped, and canoe-shaped. The straight needle has limited uses and requires a side-to-side pushing motion to advance it through tissues. The advantages of the straight needle are that it is easy to grasp and it passes easily through any port. The ski- and canoe-shaped needles also pass easily through most ports but provide a better approach to the tissue than a straight needle. Furthermore, they curve through an arc with less tension and trauma to tissue. The curved needle provides the most natural passage through the tissue but is somewhat more difficult to load onto needle drivers. Also, larger curved needles may not fit through a given port site and are more likely to get caught up on the inside of a trocar. Sutures on 2-0 or 4-0 tapered needles are most commonly used at our institution and are extracorporeally cut approximately 8 cm for intracorporeal knot tying of an interrupted suture.

The Simple Stitch

Introducing Needle and Suture Into the Body and Loading the Needle Driver

Under most circumstances, the needle and suture can be passed directly through the trocar. To pass the needle, hold the suture with a needle driver or grasper several centimeters behind the swage of the needle. Then open the trapdoor of the trocar with one hand and pass the instrument channel through the trocar, taking care not to tear rubber gasket or valve with the needle. A reducing sleeve may also help to avoid catching the needle and suture on the inner workings of the trocar but is not usually necessary. The limiting factor is the size of the needle; larger curved needles may require a 10-mm instead of a 5-mm port. The largest needles require removing the trocar and actually passing the needle through the port site incision.

Once inside the peritoneum, watch the needle at all times for safety. To grasp the needle, either hold the needle near its tip with the grasper and then grab it with the needle driver or place the needle on a flat surface and pick it up with the needle driver. A good needle driver does the following:

1. Secures the needle with a minimum of readjustment needed
2. Permits multiple angles of alignment
3. Allows wrist supination to finesse the needle through its arc
4. Grasps the suture without fraying or kinking

Self-righting needle holders make it easy to secure the needle initially but usually limit the needle angle in the jaws to 90 or 45 degrees. Newer laparoscopic needle drivers mimic standard needle drivers (Fig. 2–10). The latest laparoscopic devices provide more ergonomic, traditional operation of the needle driver. For instance, the Endopath needle holder (Ethicon Endo-Surgery) is a 5-mm device with two jaw-like handles and a magnetic, self-righting tip that automatically loads any needle at 90 degrees (Fig. 2–11). The in-line handles allow smooth, unfettered wrist supination and fit comfortably in the hand. However, unlike the release of jaws of traditional needle holders at laparotomy, with the Endopath needle holder, a button must be pressed with the index finger to release the clamped jaws. This action can be awkward when the wrist is in the maximally supinated position.

Passing the Stitch

The rule of laparoscopic suturing should be, "Place the stitch perfectly on the first pass." The time it takes to withdraw the needle, reload the needle driver, retract the tissue, and provide countertension for a misplaced stitch makes good preparation especially important in laparoscopic surgery.

With the needle in place in the driver, advance the laparoscope for a close-up of the suture site and use the grasper to present the tissue to the needle tip. As in open surgery, the tip of the needle enters perpendicular to the tissue surface, and the rest of needle gently follows through on its arc. When the tip emerges on the other side, secure it with graspers, release the

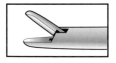

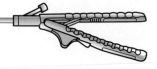

FIGURE 2–10. Standard laparoscopic needle holder (Ethicon, Cincinnati, OH).

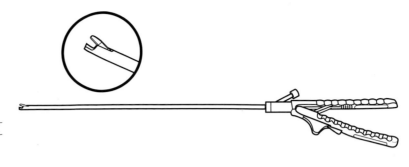

FIGURE 2–11. The Endopath needle holder (Ethicon, Cincinnati, OH) has a self-righting jaw that holds any needle at a 90-degree angle.

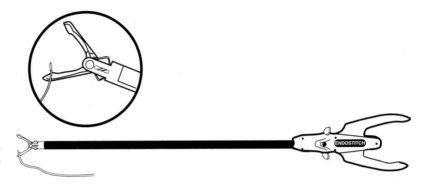

FIGURE 2–12. EndoStitch suturing device (U.S. Surgical, Norwalk, CT). *Inset,* Close-up of jaws showing T needle with suture exiting the center of the needle. The surgeon passes the needle from one jaw to the other by tilting a lever on the instrument's handle.

needle driver's jaws, and pull the needle through the rest of its arc. Grasping the needle before releasing the needle driver prevents back-slip of the needle tip into the tissue. Alternatively, instead of securing the needle with graspers, reload the needle farther back on its swage and advance it through the tissue until a decent portion of needle is showing. Then simply grab the needle with the driver to finish the stitch. This latter maneuver avoids the redundancy of grasping the needle twice and takes good advantage of the self-righting feature of many needle drivers.

EndoStitch

EndoStitch (AutoSuture, U.S. Surgical) is an easy-to-use, disposable 10-mm–port suturing device that eliminates the need for a separate needle driver and grasper (Fig. 2–12). It is particularly well suited to performing laparoscopic pyeloplasty. The two jaws of the instrument pass a straight needle with the attached suture back and forth and can be operated with one hand. First, choose the appropriate suture and load it onto the instrument. Next, place the target tissue between the jaws, and squeeze the handles of the instrument to bring the jaws together. This action passes the needle tip through the tissue and into the head of the apposing jaw. Tilt the dark-colored lever located on the handle to endow the receiving jaw with the task of holding the needle, and open the jaws to complete the stitch (see later discussion of suturing). Suture is available in braided synthetic absorbable, braided nylon, braided silk, and braided polyester and ranges in size between 0 and 4-0.

Knot Tying

Laparoscopic knotting is broadly classified as extracorporeal or intracorporeal. Numerous knots and tying techniques have been invented or adapted from other disciplines (fishermen, cowboys, otolaryngologists) for use in laparoscopic surgery. We think that the surgeon must become familiar with two or three extracorporeal knots and one or two methods of tying intracorporeal knots.

Extracorporeal knots generally place more tension on the tissue during tying and pushing of the knot than intracorporeal knots. Also, the 40 to 60 cm of suture that is dragged through the stitch in extracorporeal methods may macerate and saw apart more delicate tissues. A final drawback to extracorporeal knotting is the loss of intracorporeal CO_2 pressure. This loss can be alleviated by the placement of a finger over the trocar mouth while tying the knot. Intracorporeal knot tying is technically more difficult to master and generally requires more time. However, this method is preferred for microsurgical techniques and fine tissues.

Extracorporeal Knotting

The classic extracorporeal knot, the square knot, requires a long suture (80–120 cm). After passing the needle through the tissue, grab the suture with the needle driver just behind the needle and withdraw it from the trocar. At this point, both ends of the suture lie outside the patient's body. Form alternating half-hitches and advance them individually to the tissue with a knot thrower (Fig. 2–13). Take care to throw alternating hitches in opposite directions to ensure a true square knot. Next, secure both strands in one hand and keep tension on the free ends while advancing the pusher. Throwing a surgeon's knot on the first hitch will help maintain appropriate tissue tension while the second half-hitch is being formed. Tying multiple half-hitches at once, but advancing them one at a time (to avoid an air knot), may save time and prevent loss of CO_2.

A second popular and trustworthy extracorporeal knot is the locking Roeder slipknot (see earlier description of loop ligation and Fig. 2–8). The advantage of the Roeder knot over the square knot is that the entire knot is formed outside the body and advanced in a single throw to complete the stitch. This

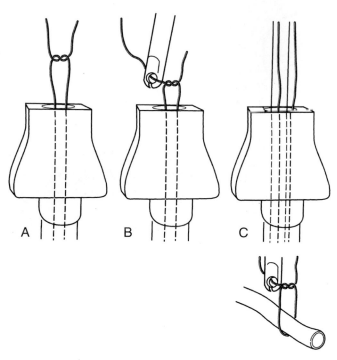

FIGURE 2–13. Tying an extracorporeal knot. *A,* Half-hitch is thrown. *B,* Both free strands are secured in one hand, and the knot pusher is used to advance the knot. *C,* While the throw is being advanced, the knot pusher applies pressure on the strand, and not directly over the knot.

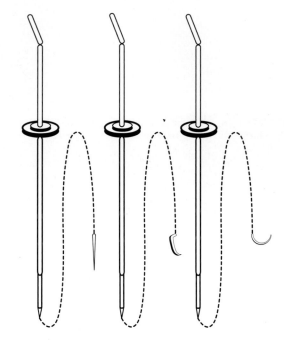

FIGURE 2–14. Surgiwip sutures (U.S. Surgical, Norwalk, CT). Three different needle configurations and suture come with a preloaded knot pusher and reducing sleeve. Once the knot is tied, the surgeon snaps the tip off the knot pusher and pulls back on the suture, while advancing the pusher to cinch the knot.

feature may be particularly useful for approximating tissues under tension. Although the standard Roeder knot takes 20 to 30 seconds to tie, the total time needed to complete the simple interrupted stitch is not longer than when using the square knot. The suture must be long enough to allow both ends to lie outside the body after the needle has been passed through the defect. First, form a simple half-hitch 4 to 6 inches above the mouth of the trocar, and pinch it between two fingers. An assistant places a finger over the trocar mouth to prevent loss of CO_2. Next, wrap one of the suture ends around the two strands several times: a minimum of three passes is required for braided and gut suture; five to seven passes are needed for monofilament suture. The knot is finished by either (1) passing the free end of the suture through the two strands and cinching it tight or (2) wrapping the free end around one of the strands and then bringing the end back up through the first loop formed below the half-hitch. Use a knot thrower to advance the knot down to the tissue, as previously described for the square knot. Another half-hitch or two can be thrown on top of this knot for maximum security.

The EndoSuture and Surgiwip (U.S. Surgical) systems simplify the knotting process by providing suture with a preloaded knot pusher. This saves the step of picking up a reusable knot pusher and positioning it on the suture. In the EndoSuture system, the small disposable knot pusher and suture are loaded onto a reusable metal handle, which then functions as the knot pusher after the knot is tied extracorporeally in the usual fashion. The Surgiwip system functions much like the Surgitie loop ligature discussed previously: The proximal tip of the plastic knot pusher is snapped off, and the attached suture is pulled to advance the knot while the knot pusher is advanced. Straight, curved, and ski-shaped needles with a variety of suture materials and sizes are available with this system (Fig. 2–14).

Intracorporeal Knotting

SQUARE KNOT. There are many variations on this basic surgeon's square knot (smiley face, triple twist, rotational [Roeder-like]), but the sequence described here suffices for most procedures. The knot is akin to the open surgical instrument tie (Fig. 2–15*A* to *D*) and needs to be part of every laparoscopic surgeon's arsenal. The ability to convert a square knot to a sliding knot is a useful skill for approximating tissues under tension (see Fig. 2–15*E* to *H*). After creating the slipknot, slide it into place on the tissue and convert it back to a square knot, then pull it tight. Add additional half-hitches to complete the knot, and cut the sutures to leave 6-mm tails.

ENDOSTITCH. After placing a simple stitch with this suturing device, as described previously, the jaws may be closed and the instrument drawn back through its 10-mm port to tie an extracorporeal knot. This approach, however, limits the surgeon to one stitch per load (about $25 to $30 per load). An intracorporeal knot is preferred for multiple interrupted stitches or a running suture line. Briefly, pass the needle between the jaws of the EndoStitch, and use a grasper to lay the free end of suture between the two jaws (Fig. 2–16*A* and *B*). Next, pass the needle back to the original jaw (see Fig. 2–16*C*), and pull the suture through the loop to create the first half-hitch (see Fig. 2–16*D* and *E*). Repeat this sequence several times to throw subsequent half-hitches and complete the knot.

Running Suture

Starting the Running Stitch

The running suture line may be started with any of the simple stitches and devices described previously, including the Endo-

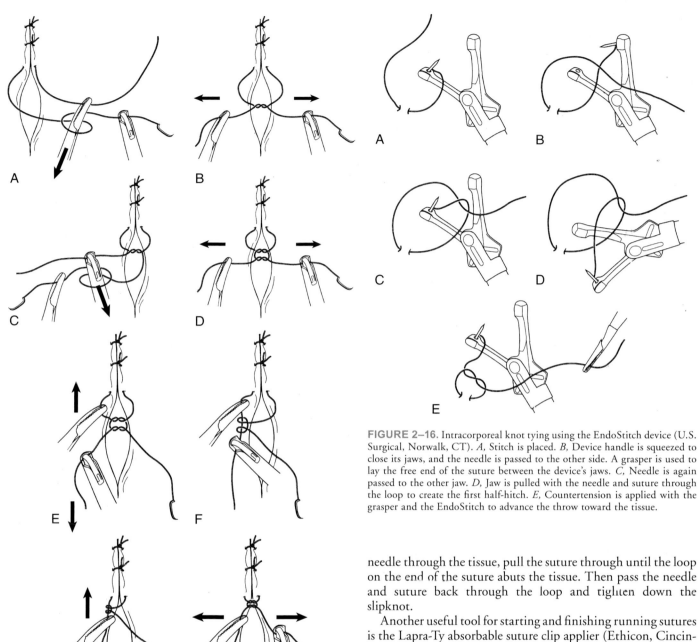

FIGURE 2–15. Intracorporeal square knot. *A–D,* Instrument tie formation of a square knot. *E–H,* Conversion of a square knot into a sliding knot. The ability to perform this conversion is useful to avoid throwing intracorporeal "air knots."

FIGURE 2–16. Intracorporeal knot tying using the EndoStitch device (U.S. Surgical, Norwalk, CT). *A,* Stitch is placed. *B,* Device handle is squeezed to close its jaws, and the needle is passed to the other side. A grasper is used to lay the free end of the suture between the device's jaws. *C,* Needle is again passed to the other jaw. *D,* Jaw is pulled with the needle and suture through the loop to create the first half-hitch. *E,* Countertension is applied with the grasper and the EndoStitch to advance the throw toward the tissue.

needle through the tissue, pull the suture through until the loop on the end of the suture abuts the tissue. Then pass the needle and suture back through the loop and tighten down the slipknot.

Another useful tool for starting and finishing running sutures is the Lapra-Ty absorbable suture clip applier (Ethicon, Cincinnati, OH) (Fig. 2–18). Instead of tying a knot, a special clip is applied to the suture, anchoring it in place. This device is reusable (nondisposable), uses a 10-mm port, and comes with clips for use with 2-0, 3-0, and 4-0 coated Vicryl suture. When choosing suture for a running stitch, allow an extra 10 to 15 mm for each stitch and 10 cm more for tying a knot at the end of the line. When sewing toward oneself, place the first stitch 2 to 3 mm distal to the defect.

Sewing

Once the first anchoring stitch is placed, place additional stitches as when closing a wound during an open procedure. The EndoStitch is well designed for this task, eliminating the cumbersome task of reloading the needle after each pass (Fig. 2–19). Locking sutures may help keep tension on the suture line. Continue stitching 2 to 3 mm past the end of the defect and then prepare to finish the running suture.

Stitch and the Suture Assistant, as long as the suture end with needle is long enough for the task. Creating a jamming loop knot (Dundee knot) on the end of a suture is another way to start a running suture line (Fig. 2–17). (A Roeder knot is also acceptable for forming an end loop but takes longer to tie in this circumstance.)

Place the needle and suture with loop into the abdomen and grasp the needle with the needle driver. After passing the

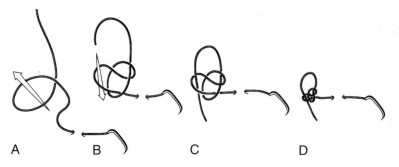

FIGURE 2–17. The jamming loop knot (Dundee knot), tied extracorporeally, is used to create a loop near the end of the suture for use in a running stitch. Make a small loop near the end of the suture *(A)* and pass a second loop through the first loop *(B)*. Next, pass the free end of suture through the second loop *(C)* and cinch tight *(D)*.

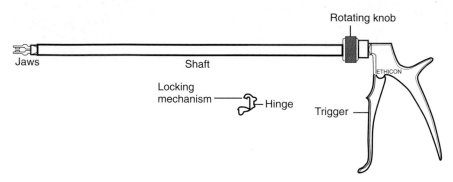

FIGURE 2–18. Lapra-Ty absorbable suture clip applier (Ethicon, Cincinnati, OH). The base unit is reusable and fits through a 10-mm port. The clip is hinged, as shown in the drawing, and locks when the handles are squeezed together.

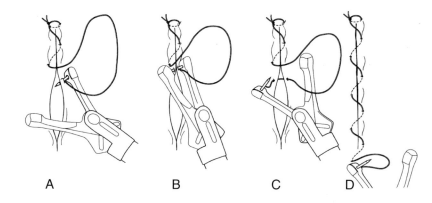

FIGURE 2–19. Running suture with the EndoStitch device (U.S. Surgical, Norwalk, CT). *A,* The first stitch is placed 2 to 3 mm distal to the defect, and the knot is placed. *B* and *C,* The needle is passed between the two jaws through the tissue to perform the actual suturing. *D,* The suture line is continued 2 to 3 mm past the end of the defect, with tension maintained on the end suture. The stitch is finished with a suture clip (see Fig. 2–20) or Aberdeen knot (see Fig. 2–21).

Terminating the Running Stitch

As previously mentioned, the Lapra-Ty absorbable clip applier was designed to place clips on suture in lieu of tying a knot. To use this instrument at the end of a running stitch, pull the free end of suture taut with a grasper and place a clip on the suture just where it exits the tissue (Fig. 2–20). Then cut the suture free, leaving an 8- to 12-mm tail, and remove the needle from the body. This method is simple, fast, and easy to learn.

The alternative to clipping the suture is tying a knot at the end. The favored knot for this purpose is the Aberdeen (Fig. 2–21) because it causes the least amount of trauma to the suture and is less likely to loosen. The Aberdeen knot is technically challenging because a fair amount of practice is required to become adept at tying the knot while maintaining tension on the suture.

LAPAROSCOPIC NEPHROPEXY

Nephropexy remains an uncommon operation yet represents a technically feasible reconstructive renal procedure for the laparoscopic surgeon. For the purpose of this chapter, nephropexy illustrates several important reconstructive techniques and requires the use of laparoscopic suturing. The use of new technology simplifies suturing of the kidney to the abdominal wall fascia.

Indications

Nephroptosis is characterized by a significant downward displacement (>5 cm) of the kidney when the patient moves from supine to erect position. The pain of nephroptosis is thought to be from either renal ischemia or renal obstruction. Symptomatic nephroptosis represents the primary clinical indication for nephropexy.

Preoperative Evaluation and Preparation

Intravenous urograms or renal scans in erect and supine positions are the best diagnostic studies for nephroptosis. Either obstruction or diminished flow to the symptomatic side is expected. Standard blood tests, chest radiograph, electrocardiogram, and oral bowel preparation with magnesium citrate are

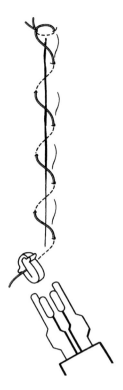

FIGURE 2–20. Lapra-Ty (Ethicon Endo-Surgery, Inc., Cincinnati, OH) used to finish a a running suture without a knot.

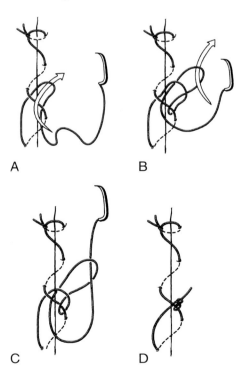

A B

C D

FIGURE 2–21. Aberdeen knot to finish a running suture.

performed the day before surgery. The patient is admitted to the hospital the day of surgery.

Patient Positioning

We prefer lateral insufflation to establish pneumoperitoneum, and we position the patient in the modified lateral position.

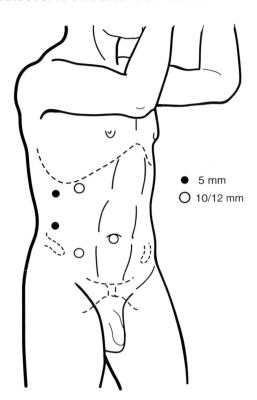

● 5 mm
○ 10/12 mm

FIGURE 2–22. Port placement and patient positioning for laparoscopic nephropexy. With the patient in lateral position, five ports are typically used: two axillary ports, two midclavicular line ports, and an umbilical port.

We typically use five laparoscopic ports when performing laparoscopic nephropexy. The camera is placed at the umbilicus, and two midclavicular line (MCL) ports and two anterior axillary line ports are used (Fig. 2–22). The port configuration may vary according to the anatomy of the patient. Typically, patients with nephroptosis are thin and have a minimum of retroperitoneal fat, a feature that usually simplifies the dissection.

Procedure

Incise the line of Toldt by means of a grasper and dissecting scissors through the MCL ports. The colon is reflected medially, exposing the kidney in the retroperitoneum. Medially retract the colon with a Jarit retractor, and stroke the colonic reflection with a closed grasper to enter and open up the correct plane.

Incise the peritoneal reflection and Gerota's fascia over the kidney anteriorly in a T configuration with the dissecting scissors and graspers through the MCL ports (Fig. 2–23A). The kidney is fully mobilized by freeing its lower, lateral, and posterior attachments with the dissecting scissors or hook electrode (see Fig. 2–23B). Use the Jarit retractor to facilitate retraction of the kidney, if needed. Take care to fulgurate all small perforating vessels, and strip the perirenal and pararenal fat from the renal capsule. These two steps will facilitate scar formation and improve fixation of the kidney.

Once cleared, the fascia overlying the quadratus lumborum and psoas muscle is easily exposed. Through the MCL ports, laparoscopically place a series of interrupted sutures between

TABLE 3–5. DIFFERENTIAL DIAGNOSIS OF HYPOTENSION IN THE PATIENT UNDERGOING LAPAROSCOPIC SURGERY

Rate/Rhythm
Bradysrhythmias: CO_2 insufflation, traction on pelvic structures
Tachydysrhythmias: sinus tachycardia and ventricular dysrhythmias

↓ Preload
Hypovolemia
Caval compression
Vasodilation
Excessive pneumoperitoneum
Abrupt change in patient position
Tension pneumothorax
Pericardial tamponade

↓ Contractility
Hypoxemia
Myocardial ischemia
Drug-induced myocardial depression
Right ventricular failure from embolic event
Acute valve dysfunction
Severe acidosis
Abrupt increase in SVR

↓ Afterload (SVR)
Drugs
Distributive mechanisms: sepsis, anaphylaxis, neurogenic, addisonian crisis, transfusion reaction
Histamine release

SVR, systemic vascular resistance.

BOX 3–1. Differential Diagnosis of Intraoperative Hypertension in the Patient Undergoing Laparoscopic Surgery

- Hypoxemia
- Hypercarbia
- Pneumoperitoneum
- Light anesthesia
- Preexisting hypertension
  - Primary
  - Renovascular
- Volume overload
- Drugs
- Elevated intracranial pressure
- Autonomic hyperreflexia
- Malignant hyperthermia
- Endocrine
  - Pheochromocytoma, carcinoid, glomus tumors, thyrotoxicosis

Courtesy of Steven G. Venticinque, MD.

the anesthetized patient undergoing laparoscopic surgery should be considered (Table 3–5) with treatment directed by the cause. Most frequently, it involves release of the pneumoperitoneum. Vasopressor agents are commonly used to temporize perfusion to the heart and brain, although they are detrimental in the setting of hypovolemic or hemorrhagic shock. Atropine is indicated for bradydysrhythmias thought to be the cause of the hypotension. While less common, hypertension may also occur; hypertension also warrants a thorough differential (Box 3–1).

TABLE 3–6. DIFFERENTIAL DIAGNOSIS OF INTRAOPERATIVE INCREASED PEAK AIRWAY PRESSURE IN THE PATIENT UNDERGOING LAPAROSCOPIC SURGERY

Anesthesia Circuit Factors
Kink
Secretions
One-way valve malfunction

Endotracheal Tube Factors
Endobronchial intubation
Secretions
Kink or patient biting on endotracheal tube

Patient Factors
Pneumoperitoneum
Bronchospasm
Mucus plug
Pneumothorax, hemothorax
Pulmonary edema
ARDS, pneumonia, aspiration
Poor baseline pulmonary compliance
    Restrictive lung disease
    Obesity
    Kyphoscoliosis

ARDS, acute respiratory distress syndrome.

Elevated Peak Airway Pressures

Functional residual capacity (FRC) and lung compliance decrease with pneumoperitoneum.[11] Several studies have documented increased peak airway pressures during pneumoperitoneum.[23,27] The peak airway pressures increase approximately 50% above baseline values.[11] Interestingly, patients with documented cardiorespiratory disease did not appear to have significant elevation in peak airway pressures beyond patients with normal cardiopulmonary status.[21] Position changes such head-up or head-down do not appreciably alter peak airway pressures.[27] Other airway misadventures must be in the differential diagnosis of increased peak airway pressure (Table 3–6). Patients with significant pulmonary disease may manifest marked elevations of $PaCO_2$ as a result of the ventilator-limiting airway pressures and in some circumstances may make maintaining a pneumoperitoneum difficult. Despite this, patients with significant pulmonary disease should not be dismissed as potential candidates for laparoscopic surgery and they may in fact benefit postoperatively. Fortunately, once the pneumoperitoneum is released the inspiratory airway pressures return to baseline.

Hypoxemia

With the institution of the pneumoperitoneum there is a drop in PaO_2. This decrease in the PaO_2 rarely results in hypoxemia in ASA (American Society of Anesthesiology physical classification) I/II patients.[11] Some reports demonstrate an increased PaO_2 when local anesthesia was used.[87] When hypoxemia occurs, many potential etiologies should be considered (Table 3–7). Baseline decreases in PaO_2 may result in more significant decreases on insufflation. Patients who require home O_2 are at high risk for hypoxemia and may require periodic release of the pneumoperitoneum. Smokers may also be more prone to hypoxemia.[88] In addition, endobronchial intubation is common during pneumoperitoneum secondary to the cephalad movement of the diaphragm.[89] Peak end-expiratory pressure may be

TABLE 3–7. DIFFERENTIAL DIAGNOSIS OF HYPOXEMIA IN THE PATIENT UNDERGOING LAPAROSCOPIC SURGERY

Hypoventilation
Esophageal intubation
Main stem intubation
Failure to ventilate
Airway obstruction
Pneumoperitoneum

V̇/Q̇ Mismatch
Main stem intubation
Atelectasis
Pulmonary edema
Bronchospasm
Aspiration
ARDS
Pneumothorax
Embolic phenomena
Shunt
　Intrapulmonary
　Intracardiac

Diminished S$\bar{v}o_2$
Shock
Decreased functional residual capacity compared with closing capacity

ARDS, acute respiratory distress syndrome.

TABLE 3–8. DIFFERENTIAL DIAGNOSIS OF OLIGURIA IN THE PATIENT UNDERGOING LAPAROSCOPIC SURGERY

Prerenal	**Postrenal**
Hypovolemia	Obstruction
Decreased cardiac output	Bladder catheter
Hypotension	Ureteral
Intrinsic	
Acute tubular necrosis	
Increased ADH	
Glomerulonephritis	

ADH, antidiuretic hormone.

of risk factors correlates with increased incidence of PONV.[97] While PONV is considered a minor complaint, it can be quite distressing to the patient and leads to increased length of stay in the ambulatory surgical center and decreased patient satisfaction.[98] Gan provided useful guidelines for prophylactic antiemetic therapy based on multimodal therapy[96] (Fig. 3–6). Other factors that may decrease PONV are stomach drainage[99] and possibly the avoidance of N_2O.[57] Nonopioid analgesics not only may be beneficial in reducing the pain after laparoscopic surgery but also may decrease PONV by minimizing postoperative opioids.

Postoperative Pain

Postoperative pain from laparoscopy is significantly less than that from laparotomy, although patients can have significant discomfort following laparoscopic procedures. Shoulder and neck pain is reported by up to 63% of patients following laparoscopic procedures.[100–102] Pain after laparoscopic surgery occurs at multiple locations and typically has a bimodal distribution. Visceral pan predominates immediately after the surgery and subsides quickly while shoulder pain can increase and not peak for up to 3 days.[103] Pain out of proportion to the procedure should prompt an investigation for possible surgical causes (e.g., hemorrhage, bladder perforation, bowel injury, nerve injury).

There are a variety of techniques used to minimize discomfort after laparoscopic procedures (Table 3–9). Many of these techniques have conflicting data regarding their efficacy. In addition, many of these techniques help with pain in the immediate postoperative period but have little effect within 24 hours. That being said, many of these techniques are safe and should be considered. The most promising technique for reduction of postoperative pain appears to be multimodal therapy whereby opioids, nonsteroidal anti-inflammatory drugs, modification of the gas, and local anesthetics are used.

There are a large variety of pharmacologic measures that can reduce postoperative pain. Opioids are effective in alleviating postsurgical discomfort. However, these drugs, in larger doses, have side effects, making their use less desirable (e.g., PONV, sedation, respiratory depression). Other analgesics that can be considered include tramadol and acetaminophen. Nonsteroidal anti-inflammatory drugs have a role for postoperative pain, although it is probably not as great as previously thought.[100,101] More novel pharmacologic measures have been investigated; one of these is low-dose ketamine. Ketamine as an analgesic adjunct has been shown to reduce postoperative pain and opioid requirements and the incidence of residual pain until the sixth

useful in increasing mean airway pressure, which may improve oxygenation. The immediate treatment of hypoxemia involves increasing the delivered O_2 to the patient. Some surgeons advocate an FIO_2 of greater than 50% to provide an added margin of safety during insufflation.

Oliguria

Decreased urine output is a common complication of pneumoperitoneum and pneumoretroperitoneum.[90] The mechanism for the decreased urine output cannot simply be explained by decreased venous return with subsequent decreased cardiac output.[91,92] If this were the only factor, then expansion of the blood volume should improve urine output. Animal studies have demonstrated that extrarenal pressures as little as 10 mm Hg impair renal blood flow and urine production.[92,93] Neurohormonal factors play a role in the decreased urine output observed clinically. Pneumoperitoneum increases plasma renin and ADH levels.[90] One study found warm insufflating CO_2 to be associated with greater urine output.[94]

Anesthetic drugs also decrease renal blood flow, GFR, and urine output.[95] The decrease in urine output due to anesthetic-related effects can be attenuated by perioperative hydration.[91,92] Once the pneumoperitoneum or pneumoretroperitoneum is deflated, an increase in urine output should follow. If prompt improvement of urine output does not occur, a thorough search for other etiologies should be conducted (Table 3–8).

POSTOPERATIVE MANAGEMENT

Nausea and Emesis

PONV is one of the most frequent complaints following laparoscopic procedures. Risks for PONV include laparoscopic surgery, female gender, history of PONV or motion sickness, postoperative opioid use, and nonsmoker.[96] Increased number

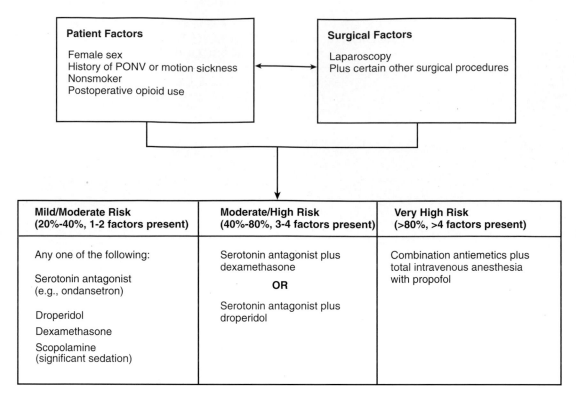

FIGURE 3–6. Treatment strategies for the prophylaxis of postoperative nausea and vomiting. (Adapted from Gan TJ: Postoperative nausea and vomiting—Can it be eliminated? JAMA 287:1233–1236, 2002.)

TABLE 3–9. ANALGESIC STRATEGIES FOR PATIENT UNDERGOING LAPAROSCOPIC SURGERY

Pharmacologic
Opioids
NSAIDs
Acetaminophen
Acetazolamide
Ketamine

Wound Bed Manipulation
Subcutaneous local anesthetic
Intra-abdominal local anesthetic
Intra-abdominal saline

Manipulation of Insufflation Gas
Heating
Humidification
Aspiration of gas
Low-pressure insufflation
Low-flow insufflation

month.[104] Use of ketamine with major renal surgery also showed a decrease in postoperative analgesic requirements.[105] Even acetazolamide has been given with modest success in reduction of referred pain in the immediate postoperative period.[106]

Local anesthetics have been looked at to relieve postoperative pain, again with varying success. Local anesthetics have been infiltrated both at and in the port sites. These interventions appear to provide brief relief[101]; interestingly, even the instillation of a relatively large volume of normal saline confers some benefit.[107] In addition to agents, there are interventions that can be done involving the insufflating gas; removal of the gas has shown minimal effect, whereas heating of the insufflating gas has the ability to produce a prolonged reduction in pain.[102]

Low-pressure insufflation also appears to offer similar advantages as heated gases.[101,108]

Pulmonary Impairment

Postoperative pulmonary complications (PPCs) are an important area of morbidity and mortality in clinical medicine. PPCs comprise a group of events such as pneumonia, respiratory failure, bronchospasm, atelectasis, and hypoxemia.[109] Risk factors for PPCs include surgery lasting longer than 3 hours, general anesthesia, upper abdominal surgery or thoracic surgery, and intraoperative use of pancuronium.[110] Potential patient-related risk factors include smoking, ASA class greater than II, age older than 70 years, obesity, obstructive sleep apnea, and COPD.[110] The risk of PPCs is lower in patients who undergo laparoscopic cholecystectomy than those undergoing open cholecystectomy.[110] There are a multitude of studies showing improved postoperative pulmonary function when comparing laparoscopy with laparotomy.[25] Strategies to improve postoperative pulmonary function have been outlined elsewhere.[109,110]

SUMMARY

Minimally invasive urologic surgery is increasingly common. Postoperative benefits include less pain, shorter hospital stay, and better postoperative pulmonary function. As more procedures are performed laparoscopically, the anesthesiologist and urologist need to understand the unique physiologic events that occur as a result of laparoscopy. For the healthy patient undergoing laparoscopy, the cardiorespiratory events are usually little more than minor intraoperative issues. However, for the patient with cardiac or pulmonary compromise, the physiologic perturbation can be more severe and requires more preoperative planning.

Tips and Tricks

- It is important to avoid and recognize the adverse physiologic affects associated with laparoscopic surgery.
- The capnograph is a useful tool to diagnose and differentiate causes of adverse affects associated with CO_2 insufflation.
- The surgery team, including operative nurses and anesthesia providers, should routinely discuss and rehearse the management and therapy of severe adverse affects related to positioning, increased intra-abdominal pressure, and CO_2 insufflation.
- Multimodality therapy for the prophylaxis of postoperative nausea and vomiting as well as postoperative pain can decrease patient discomfort and improve patient satisfaction with minimally invasive surgery.

REFERENCES

1. Joshi GP: Complications of laparoscopy. Anesthesiol Clin North Am 19:89–105, 2001.
2. Guller U, Hervey S, Purves H, et al: Laparoscopic versus open appendectomy: Outcomes comparison based on a large administrative database. Ann Surg 239:43–52, 2004.
3. Memon MA, Cooper NJ, Memon B, et al: Meta-analysis of randomized clinical trials comparing open and laparoscopic inguinal hernia repair. Br J Surg 90:1479–1492, 2003.
4. Guller U, Jain N, Hervey S, et al: Laparoscopic vs open colectomy: Outcomes comparison based on large nationwide databases. Arch Surg 138:1179–1186, 2003.
5. Johnson N, Barlow D, Lethaby A, et al: Methods of hysterectomy: Systematic review and meta-analysis of randomised controlled trials. BMJ 330:1478, 2005.
6. Sauerland S, Lefering R, Neugebauer EA: Laparoscopic versus open surgery for suspected appendicitis. [Update in Cochrane Database Syst Rev 2004(4):CD001546.PMID:15495014]. Cochrane Database Syst Rev CD001546, 2002.
7. Fahlenkamp D, Rassweiler J, Fornara P, et al: Complications of laparoscopic procedures in urology: Experience with 2,407 procedures at 4 German centers. J Urol 162:765–770, discussion 770–771, 1999.
8. Sundqvist P, Feuk U, Haggman M, et al: Hand-assisted retroperitoneoscopic live donor nephrectomy in comparison to open and laparoscopic procedures: A prospective study on donor morbidity and kidney function. Transplantation 78:147–153, 2004.
9. Le Blanc-Louvry I, Coquerel A, Koning E, et al: Operative stress response is reduced after laparoscopic compared to open cholecystectomy: The relationship with postoperative pain and ileus. Dig Dis Sci 45:1703–1713, 2000.
10. Schauer PR, Sirinek KR: The laparoscopic approach reduces the endocrine response to elective cholecystectomy. Am Surg 61:106–111, 1995.
11. O'Malley C, Cunningham AJ: Physiologic changes during laparoscopy. Anesthesiol Clin North Am 19:1–9, 2001.
12. Rose DK, Cohen MM, Soutter DI: Laparoscopic cholecystectomy: The anaesthetist's point of view. Can J Anaesth 39:809–815, 1992.
13. Deziel DJ, Millikan KW, Economou SG, et al: Complications of laparoscopic cholecystectomy: A national survey of 4,292 hospitals and an analysis of 77,604 cases. Am J Surg 165:9–14, 1993.
14. Hemal AK, Kumar R, Seth A, et al: Complications of laparoscopic radical cystectomy during the initial experience. Int J Urol 11:483–488, 2004.
15. Gill IS, Kavoussi LR, Clayman RV, et al: Complications of laparoscopic nephrectomy in 185 patients: A multi-institutional review. J Urol 154:479–483, 1995.
16. Kavoussi LR, Sosa E, Chandhoke P, et al: Complications of laparoscopic pelvic lymph node dissection. J Urol 149:322–325, 1993.
17. Mertens zur Borg IR, Lim A, Verbrugge SJ, et al: Effect of intraabdominal pressure elevation and positioning on hemodynamic responses during carbon dioxide pneumoperitoneum for laparoscopic donor nephrectomy: A prospective controlled clinical study. Surg Endosc 18:919–923, 2004.
18. Meininger D, Byhahn C, Bueck M, et al: Effects of prolonged pneumoperitoneum on hemodynamics and acid-base balance during totally endoscopic robot-assisted radical prostatectomies. World J Surg 26:1423–1427, 2002.
19. Nguyen NT, Ho HS, Fleming NW, et al: Cardiac function during laparoscopic vs open gastric bypass. Surg Endosc 16:78–83, 2002.
20. Menes T, Spivak H: Laparoscopy: Searching for the proper insufflation gas. Surg Endosc 14:1050–1056, 2000.
21. Wittgen CM, Andrus CH, Fitzgerald SD, et al: Analysis of the hemodynamic and ventilatory effects of laparoscopic cholecystectomy. Arch Surg 126:997–1000; discussion 1000–1001, 1991.
22. Motew M, Ivankovich AD, Bieniarz J, et al: Cardiovascular effects and acid-base and blood gas changes during laparoscopy. Am J Obstet Gynecol 115:1002–1012, 1973.
23. Hardacre JM, Talamini MA: Pulmonary and hemodynamic changes during laparoscopy—Are they important? Surgery 127:241–244, 2000.
24. Girardis M, Broi UD, Antonutto G, et al: The effect of laparoscopic cholecystectomy on cardiovascular function and pulmonary gas exchange. Anesth Analg 83:134–140, 1996.
25. Joris J: Anesthesia for laparoscopic surgery. In Miller RD (ed): Miller's Anesthesia, 6th ed. Philadelphia, Churchill Livingstone, 2005, pp 22–93.
26. Ortega AE, Richman MF, Hernandez M, et al: Inferior vena caval blood flow and cardiac hemodynamics during carbon dioxide pneumoperitoneum. Surg Endosc 10:920, 1996.
27. Rauh R, Hemmerling TM, Rist M, et al: Influence of pneumoperitoneum and patient positioning on respiratory system compliance. J Clin Anesth 13:361–365, 2001.
28. Fujise K, Shingu K, Matsumoto S, et al: The effects of the lateral position on cardiopulmonary function during laparoscopic urological surgery. Anesth Analg 87:925–930, 1998.
29. Sprung J, Whalley DG, Falcone T, et al: The impact of morbid obesity, pneumoperitoneum, and posture on respiratory system mechanics and oxygenation during laparoscopy. Anesth Analg 94:1345–1350, 2002.
30. Moncure M, Salem R, Moncure K, et al: Central nervous system metabolic and physiologic effects of laparoscopy. Am Surg 65:168–172, 1999.
31. Fernandez-Cruz L, Saenz A, Taura P, et al: Helium and carbon dioxide pneumoperitoneum in patients with pheochromocytoma undergoing laparoscopic adrenalectomy. World J Surg 22:1250–1255, 1998.
32. Wolf JS Jr, Clayman RV, McDougall EM, et al: Carbon dioxide and helium insufflation during laparoscopic radical nephrectomy in a patient with severe pulmonary disease. J Urol 155:20–21, 1996.
33. Eagle KA, Berger PB, Calkins H, et al: ACC/AHA guideline update for perioperative cardiovascular evaluation for noncardiac surgery—Executive summary. A report of the American College of Cardiology/American Heart Association Task Force on Practice Guidelines (Committee to Update the 1996 Guidelines on Perioperative Cardiovascular Evaluation for Noncardiac Surgery). Anesth Analg 94:1052–1064, 2002.
34. Gibby GL: How preoperative assessment programs can be justified financially to hospital administrators. Int Anesthesiol Clin 40:17–30, 2002.
35. Anonymous: Practice guidelines for preoperative fasting and the use of pharmacologic agents to reduce the risk of pulmonary aspiration: Application to healthy patients undergoing elective procedures: A report by the American Society of Anesthesiologist Task Force on Preoperative Fasting. Anesthesiology 90:896–905, 1999.
36. Sprung J, O'Hara JF Jr, Gill IS, et al: Anesthetic aspects of laparoscopic and open adrenalectomy for pheochromocytoma. Urology 55:339–343, 2000.
37. Joris JL, Hamoir EE, Hartstein GM, et al: Hemodynamic changes and catecholamine release during laparoscopic adrenalectomy for pheochromocytoma. Anesth Analg 88:16–21, 1999.
38. Wahba RW, Tessler MJ: Misleading end-tidal CO2 tensions. Can J Anaesth 43:862–866, 1996.
39. Portera CA, Compton RP, Walters DN, et al: Benefits of pulmonary artery catheter and transesophageal echocardiographic monitoring in laparoscopic cholecystectomy patients with cardiac disease. Am J Surg 169:202–206; discussion 206–207, 1995.

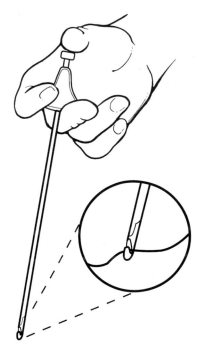

FIGURE 4–3. EndoClose suturing device (U.S. Surgical, Norwalk, CT). The spring-loaded stylet has a retractable hook that can grasp a suture when the top button is depressed. The EndoClose is inserted through one side of the incision, incorporating fascia. Depressing the top button releases the loop of suture. The EndoClose is reinserted (without suture) on the opposite side of the incision, incorporating the fascia. The notched end of the stylet is exposed, hooking the looped end of suture. Once the suture is hooked, the top button is released; the tip is thereupon drawn into the stylet and the suture is anchored. Then, the entire device is withdrawn above skin. A standard knot is tied.

obturator (Fig. 4–3). Release the button, drawing the hook and anchoring the suture at the tip of the device. Insert the Endo-Close through one side of the incision, into the peritoneum, and then depress the button to drop the suture. A grasper placed through a second port can be employed to pull the suture farther down into the incision. Externally tag the ends of the suture to prevent tangling and to maintain orientation. Then reinsert the EndoClose device on the opposite side of the incision, through the fascia, and depress the button to expose the notched end of the stylet. Use the notched end to hook the loop of suture and draw it through the incision, making a standard hand-tied knot to finish the fascial closure.

J HOOK CLOSURE DEVICE

The J Hook closure device (Advanced Surgical, Princeton, NJ) is no longer readily available but may be found in some laparoscopic instrument sets. This instrument is constructed with a needle shaped like a fishing hook that rotates 180 degrees away from the shaft of the instrument.

Pass the J Hook into the 10-mm trocar site under direct vision; when the needle swings out, withdraw the device from the trocar. This action causes the needle tip with the suture eyelet to pierce the fascia. Load the suture into the eyelet, and reinsert the device. Rotate the needle handle 180 degrees to complete passage of the suture. Remove the trocar and J Hook devices and tie the sutures.

RADIALLY EXPANDING TROCARS

Radially expanding trocars (Step, Innerdyne, Sunnyvale, CA) represent a category of nonbladed trocars that develop incisions parallel to muscle fibers and a narrower tract. This blunt effect of the trocar placement results in not having to close the fascia even in incisions up to 12 mm.[4] Place the trocar by first applying an expandable mesh sleeve trocar over a Veress needle (Fig. 4–4A). Subsequently, pass a blunt-tipped fascial dilator through the mesh sleeve lumen (see Fig. 4–4B). Use the nondominant hand to stabilize the trocar with upward traction on the mesh sleeve while the fascial dilator and sheath are inserted. Use caution in placing these trocars because nonbladed trocars require more force for insertion.

FINAL SURVEY

After every laparoscopic procedure, conduct a careful and complete survey of the operative field. This is necessary to inspect for bleeding and unrecognized injury. Lower the pneumoperitoneum to a pressure of less than 5 mm Hg for 5 to 10 minutes to allow visualization of bleeding vessels that may have been occluded by higher working pressures during the procedure. Significant venous bleeding can occur once the abdominal pressure has been lowered to less than 5 mm Hg. Inspect the entire operative field to identify any previously unrecognized injury.

Use irrigation in an orderly and systematic fashion, if necessary, to wash the field for final inspection. Yellow or brown returned irrigation fluid may be a sign of an unrecognized bowel injury. Incisions larger than 5 mm require fascial closure in all patients in order to prevent bowel herniation. In children, close port sites smaller than 5 mm.

SEQUENCE OF TROCAR REMOVAL

Removal of the trocars using a specific routine each time is done for a few reasons:

1. Ensure adequate closure of the trocar sites
2. Assist with evacuation of the pneumoperitoneum
3. Possibly shorten the procedure time

The following sequence is recommended.

First, place all the fascial sutures at the 10/12-mm trocar sites. Initially, do not tie the sutures and re-place the trocars into the abdomen to maintain pressure for adequate visualization during closure and evacuation of the pneumoperitoneum. Remove the 5-mm trocars under direct vision, and inspect the sites under laparoscopic control for bleeding. Next, sequentially remove 10/12-mm trocar sites other than the camera site under direct vision, and tie the fascial sutures. Escaping gas from a

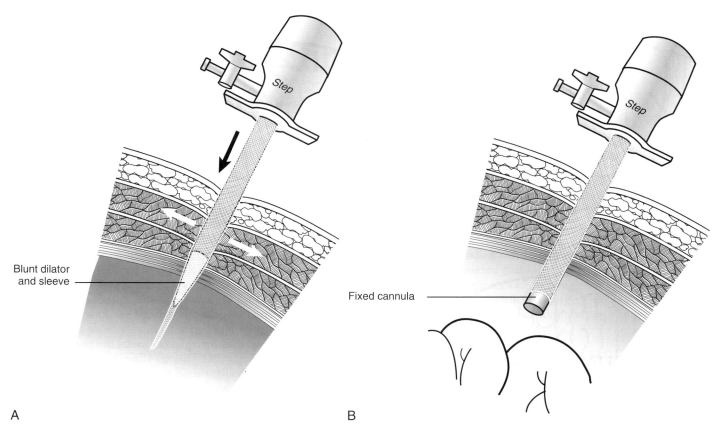

A

B

FIGURE 4–4. Radially expanding blunt-tipped trocar. *A,* First the expandable mesh sleeve trocar with Veress needle is inserted. Next, a blunt-tipped fascial dilator back-loaded with a trocar is inserted. *B,* Upward traction on the sleeve results in minimal downward traction of the abdominal wall during dilation. These trocars do not require fascial closure upon removal.

10/12-mm trocar site may indicate the need for additional sutures.

It is important that as much of the pneumoperitoneum be evacuated as possible before removal of the last trocar. When CO_2 is used as an insufflation agent, it is metabolized to carbonic acid and water on the peritoneal surface. Carbonic acid may cause diaphragmatic irritation, leading to postoperative shoulder, chest, or back pain. Residual pneumoscrotum or subcutaneous emphysema usually resolves within 24 to 48 hours.

Direct the last 10/12-mm trocar with the camera to the highest portion of the abdomen or working space, which harbors the greatest amount of gas (Fig. 4–5). Turn off the CO_2 and disconnect it from the trocar; make sure the trocar insufflation valve is in the open position to allow gas to escape. Apply external, manual pressure to the abdomen to help direct the gas to the trocar, evacuating a larger amount of intra-abdominal gas. In addition, the anesthesia team can use manual ventilation to assist in maximizing gas evacuation from the abdomen.

Pull up the previously placed fascial sutures to place tension on the wound edges; this maneuver will prevent herniation as the trocar and endoscope are removed. First, back out the trocar from the abdomen over the lens, leaving only the laparoscope in the abdomen. Then slowly remove the laparoscope, allowing inspection of the trocar tract for bleeding as the laparoscope is moved. Then secure the final fascial suture.

SKIN CLOSURE

Irrigate the trocar site and achieve adequate hemostasis of the skin edges before skin closure. After fascial closure, suture the skin with a subcuticular suture of 4-0 Vicryl on a cutting needle. Stapling is possible, although a better cosmetic result is obtained with a subcuticular suture.

SUMMARY

Closure of the abdominal cavity, inspection of the surgical field, and evacuation of residual CO_2 are important steps in every laparoscopic procedure. Trocar sites larger than 5 mm need to be closed in all patients. Closure of the fascia prevents herniation of omentum and abdominal viscera and dehiscence of wounds.[5] Patient habitus and laterally placed trocars may produce a difficult open closure. Therefore, it is important to be familiar with alternative techniques for closure.

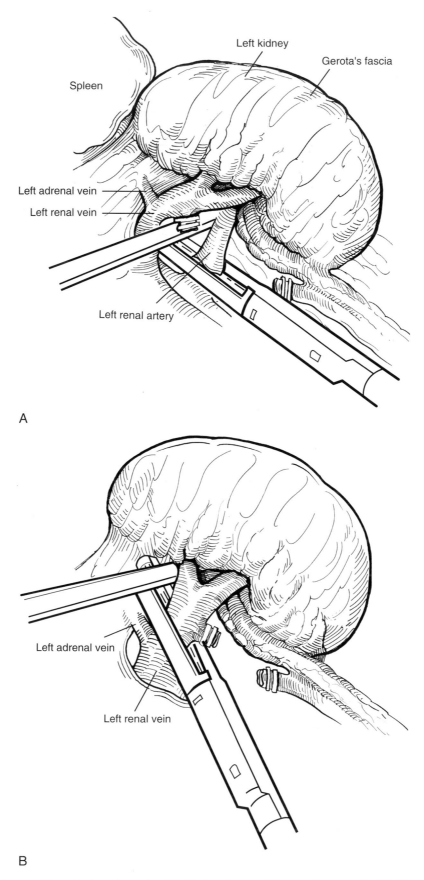

A

B

FIGURE 5–6. *A,* The artery is stapled first with the endovascular GIA. During this part of the procedure it may be helpful to place the retracting instrument between the renal artery and vein. This will provide more arterial length and separate artery from vein. *B,* The renal vein is ligated lateral to the adrenal vein with the endovascular GIA. During a simple nephrectomy, it is often possible to divide the renal vein lateral to the gonadal vein, leaving both the gonadal and adrenal veins intact.

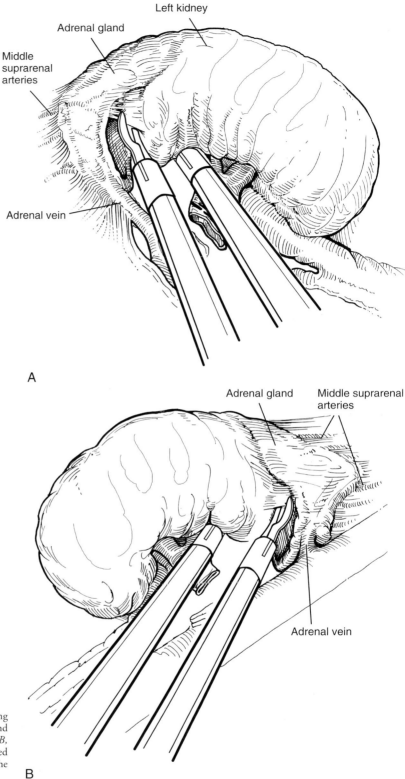

FIGURE 5–7. *A,* The left adrenal gland can be preserved during simple nephrectomy. Here, the left renal vein has been preserved and the dissection is continued directly on the capsule of the kidney. *B,* Preservation of the right adrenal gland. Caution must be exercised on the right so as not to avulse the short right adrenal vein from the vena cava.

Left-Sided Procedures

Superior pole dissection on the left side often poses greater challenges to the surgeon than right-sided procedures. The spleen, pancreas, adrenal gland, colon, and diaphragm are in intimate relation to the left kidney. The plane of dissection must proceed immediately adjacent to the upper pole of the

kidney. The harmonic scalpel and a liberal amount of clips help in this dissection because problematic bleeding can be encountered in this region. Any retraction of the spleen must be gentle and superomedial. Retract the spleen only after adequate ligation of lienorenal attachments in order to prevent tearing of the delicate splenic capsule. Furthermore, it is important to dissect lateral to the spleen in a superior direction so that the spleen

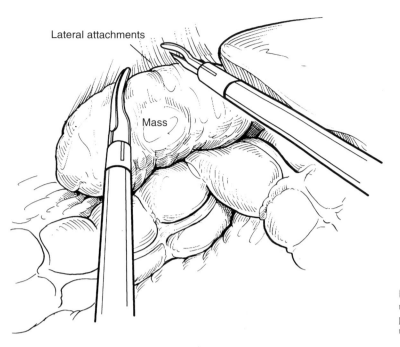

FIGURE 6–15. The lateral attachments to the side wall and the posterior attachments to the psoas muscle are divided. The kidney is pulled medially, and electrocautery, scissors, or blunt dissection with the tip of the irrigator-aspirator is used to free the kidney.

Dividing the Ureter

If not already divided during upper and lateral pole dissection, now divide the ureter between clips. Do not divide the ureter before securing the renal hilum because the ureter gives stability to the specimen and provides anatomic orientation during hilar dissection.

Observing for Hemostasis

After the specimen is completely freed in the abdominal cavity, use graspers to move the kidney from the renal fossa by placing it above the liver or spleen. Lower the pneumoperitoneum to a pressure of 5 mm Hg or less for at least 5 minutes. Closely observe the entire operative field and especially the renal hilum to find any vessels that may have been occluded by higher pressures during the procedure. Address any unrecognized bleeding or injury at this time.

Entrapping the Specimen

Perform intra-abdominal entrapment of the excised specimen to facilitate removal. If the specimen is to be removed intact through an incision, use an EndoCatch retrieval device and bag (U.S. Surgical, Norwalk, CT) or similar device. The Endo-Catch instrument consists of a plastic sac attached to a self-opening, flexible metal ring. The primary advantage of a self-opening bag is that the specimen can be easily manipulated into the opening of the bag with a single grasper. The Endo-Catch comes in two sizes: 10-mm with a 6-inch-deep bag and 15-mm with a 9-inch-deep bag. The 15-mm device is usually needed for radical nephrectomy specimens and is passed directly through the skin after the 10/12-mm trocar is removed.

Before removal of the trocar, insertion of the EndoCatch device, and entrapment of the specimen, preplace fascia-closing sutures in the 10/12-mm ports under direct vision using a fascial closure device. If a radially dilating trocar device was used for port placement, fascial port closure may be unnecessary and this step can be omitted.

To entrap the specimen, position the laparoscope in the lower quadrant (10/12-mm) port and replace the umbilical trocar with the EndoCatch device. To place the 15-mm bag, remove the trocar and pass the device directly through the incision. Then lift the kidney with a 5-mm grasper, place it above the liver or spleen, open the EndoCatch bag, and carefully drop the specimen into the bag (Fig. 6–16). First, pull the drawstring to close the bag and separate it from the wire deployment ring. Next, close the ring under direct vision to ensure that trocars or vital structures are not inadvertently included in the device.

Once the specimen is in the EndoCatch bag, withdraw the EndoCatch device and bag through the trocar site (Fig. 6–17A). Cut the suture and release the device from the bag (see Fig. 6–17B). Make A 4- to 6-cm skin incision to extract the bag and specimen, and divide the fascia with electrocautery. During this maneuver, protect the specimen and bag with the index finger positioned alongside the specimen through the trocar site (see Fig. 6–17C).

Alternatively, remove the kidney through a Pfannenstiel incision. First place the EndoCatch device and bag through an incision a few centimeters above the pubis. Remove the bag and specimen through the Pfannenstiel incision (Fig. 6–18).

Most surgeons prefer intact extraction of radical nephrectomy specimens, but morcellation is an option. If the specimen is to be morcellated, the EndoCatch bag will *not* suffice because the bag's material will easily perforate during morcellation. The LapSac entrapment bag (Cook Urological, Inc., Spencer, IN) is recommended. It is fabricated from a double layer of plastic and nondistensible nylon and has been shown to be impermeable to bacteria and tumor cells.[4] This bag is not attached to any ring or instrument. Entrap the drawstring within the bag while wrapping the bag around the shaft of the laparoscopic forceps. Then introduce the bag into the abdomen through the lower quadrant port site. Remove the trocar and pass the LapSac

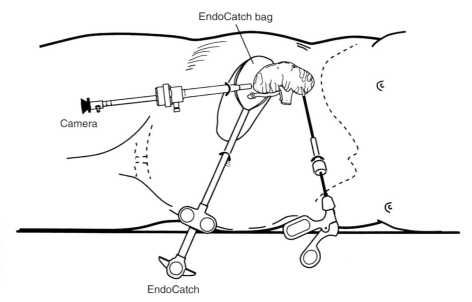

FIGURE 6–16. Placement of the specimen into an opened EndoCatch device placed through umbilical trocar site. Note that the camera is positioned in the lateral port and the specimen is maneuvered with the upper midline trocar. The umbilical trocar is removed to accommodate the 15-mm EndoCatch device.

directly through the abdominal wall (Fig. 6–19). Place the kidney above the spleen or liver before introducing the bag into the abdomen. Once the bag is in the abdominal cavity, replace the trocar by means of a blunt obturator.

After introducing the LapSac, unfurl it within the abdomen and position it flat with its bottom in the pelvis. This positioning is critical to facilitate entrapment of the specimen. Hold the bag open below the corresponding liver or spleen edge so that the specimen can be advanced slowly over the spleen or liver edge and into the open LapSac. Placing the specimen within the LapSac is often challenging, especially when there are only two ports through which to work. An additional 3- or 5-mm lateral trocar and grasper may be helpful in keeping the sac open (Fig. 6–20). Use only atraumatic graspers to manipulate the bag in order to prevent perforation. Once the specimen is inside the LapSac, grasp the drawstring, tighten it, and withdraw it into the 10-mm umbilical port, which pulls the neck of the bag into the port as well. Use of the LapSac can be facilitated by looping a hydrophilic wire through the holes in the mouth of the sac before placement in the abdomen. The loop of wire helps to hold the LapSac in the open position for easier organ entrapment (Fig. 6–21).

Removing the Specimen

If the specimen is removed intact (the preferred technique) within the EndoCatch bag, make a 4- to 6-cm periumbilical incision that incorporates the umbilical port incision or Pfannenstiel incision (see Fig. 6–17C). To aid in cosmesis, hide at least 2 cm of the incision within the umbilical fold. It is critical to take care to avoid tearing or perforating the EndoCatch bag during this step. Open the fascia and deliver the specimen.

If the specimen is to be morcellated, pull the LapSac drawstring through the umbilical port, drawing the neck of the sac into the sheath. Then remove the sheath so that the neck of the sac rests on the abdomen. Preserve the pneumoperitoneum throughout the morcellation process so that the intra-abdominal portion of the bag can be monitored laparoscopically for possible perforation. Tightly pull the sac against the abdomen, and begin morcellation. Place surgical towels around the sac,

and cover the entire surgical field to prevent contamination of the port site with any spillage of the morcellated specimen.

Morcellation can be performed either manually or with a high-speed electrical morcellator. If the electrical tissue morcellator is available, connect it to wall suction with the foot pedal. Electrical morcellators generally consist of a tissue-trapping chamber and a 10-mm barrel that contains a recessed blade. Morcellators must be used with great care. With the neck of the sac pulled tightly upward, introduce the barrel into the sac and move it back and forth through the renal tissue (Fig. 6–22A). When specimen contact is made, turn on the suction and activate the recessed blade with the foot pedal. Every few minutes, empty the aspirated renal fragments from the trapping chamber to ensure that maximum suction is maintained. To prevent aspiration and perforation of the sac, keep in mind the following points:

- Keep constant upward traction on the sac.
- Maintain continuous laparoscopic visualization of the sac.
- Use short, controlled, back-and-forth motions of the morcellator.

Alternating between electrical and manual morcellation is common and facilitates removal of fibrous fragments. The electrical morcellator alone is not effective with fibrotic kidneys.

For manual morcellation, introduce a Kelley clamp or ring forceps into the sac to fragment the kidney (see Fig. 6–22B). Systematically pull pieces of renal tissue from the sac until the residual mass is small enough to be withdrawn through the port incision. Then withdraw the bag with the residual specimen and reintroduce a 10-mm trocar to preserve the pneumoperitoneum (see Fig. 6–22C).

Closing

If the specimen is removed intact, inspect the bowel and retroperitoneum for potential bleeding or injury at both 5 and 15 mm Hg pressure before removing the specimen (see earlier). Place fascial closure sutures as necessary at the 10/12-mm trocar sites and sequentially remove the ports under

Tips and Tricks

- Be sure that the patient is positioned properly and well secured before beginning procedure.
- Use rotation of the surgical table and gravity to your advantage.
- Insert additional 5-mm ports as needed throughout the duration of the surgery with little effect on cosmesis or postoperative pain.
- Always have the tips of the scissors visible during use of electrocautery to avoid bowel injury.
- The ureter is useful for retraction during dissection of the hilum and should not be divided until the renal vessels have been divided.
- Always ensure that the stapler is completely across the vessel being divided and always be prepared for equipment malfunction.
- Upper pole dissection can be tedious but must be done with care to avoid bleeding complications and need for conversion.
- Perform meticulous closure of the extraction site fascial incision to prevent postoperative hernias.

REFERENCES

1. Finelli A, Kaouk JH, Fergany AF, et al: Laparoscopic cytoreductive nephrectomy for metastatic renal cell carcinoma. BJU Int 94:291–294, 2004.
2. Clayman RV, Kavoussi LR, Soper NJ, et al: Laparoscopic nephrectomy: Initial case report. J Urol 146:278–282, 1991.
3. Ogan, K, Cadeddu JA, Stifelman, MD: Laparoscopic radical nephrectomy: Oncological efficacy. Urol Clin N Am 30:543–550, 2003.
4. Urban DA, Kerbl K, McDougall EM, et al: Organ entrapment and renal morcellation: Permeability studies. J Urol 150:1792–1794, 1993.
5. Cadeddu JA, Ono Y, Clayman RV, et al: Laparoscopic nephrectomy for renal cell cancer: Evaluation of efficacy and safety: A multi-center experience. Urology 52:773–777, 1998.
6. Gill IS, Meraney AM, Schweizer DK, et al: Laparoscopic radical nephrectomy in 100 patients: A single center experience from the United States. Cancer 92:1843–1855, 2001.

Hand-Assisted Laparoscopic Radical Nephrectomy

George K. Chow

Hand-assisted laparoscopic radical nephrectomy (HALRN) was first described by Tierney and colleagues in 1994.[1] Although no actual hand port device was used, the kidney was extracted manually through an incision. The first reported clinical usage of a dedicated hand-assistance device for laparoscopic nephrectomy was performed by Wolf and colleagues in 1997.[2]

INDICATIONS AND CONTRAINDICATIONS

HALRN is appropriate whenever extirpative nephrectomy with intact extraction is indicated. If benign renal pathology is anticipated and morcellation will be used, pure laparoscopy would be preferable. For laparoscopists who prefer to morcellate malignant lesions, hand-assistance would also be moot.

The absolute contraindications to HALRN are renal vein or vena caval thrombus and bleeding diathesis. Another absolute contraindication is stage T4 disease with invasion into surrounding organs. The only exception to this is adrenal invasion; patients with adrenal invasion can be handled effectively by radical nephrectomy. If the patient has significant cardiopulmonary comorbidity, surgery may not be advisable. In this sense, the contraindications are not any different from those for pure laparoscopy.

Although tumor and specimen size is often considered a relative contraindication for pure laparoscopy, I find that this is less of a consideration with hand-assisted surgery. Manual assistance for retraction and dissection often facilitates removal of the large specimen.

Morbid obesity is a relative contraindication for laparoscopy. Usually, the obstacles presented by patient habitus can be overcome by modifying the hand port incision and trocar placement. I will typically place the hand port incision in a more cephalad paramedian position rather than at my typical infraumbilical site. These incisions tend to go through the rectus sheath, and one must be careful not to injure the epigastric vessels. An additional caveat is that both the anterior and posterior rectus sheaths need to be closed. Closing the anterior sheath alone is insufficient, and bowel herniation into the rectus sheath can occur.

PATIENT PREOPERATIVE EVALUATION AND PREPARATION

As with all radical nephrectomy patients, careful preoperative metastatic work-up is necessary. Order chest radiography or chest computed tomography (CT) to evaluate the chest for metastatic disease. Cross-sectional imaging of the abdomen with CT or magnetic resonance imaging (MRI) is useful to determine presence of metastatic disease or invasion of contiguous organs. The additional benefit of cross-sectional abdominal imaging is that vascular anomalies such as multiple vessels can be identified preoperatively, facilitating surgery. MRI is especially useful for ruling out tumor thrombus. If the patient has unexplained bone pain, order a bone scan. Furthermore, if the patient manifests neurologic signs or symptoms, order CT of the head.

Carefully evaluate the patient medically for anesthetic risk factors. Also, address any other conditions that may affect surgery such as cessation of anticoagulant therapy, subacute bacterial endocarditis prophylaxis, and potential drug allergies.

The day before surgery, instruct the patient to take a liquid dinner and stop eating and drinking after midnight. A light laxative preparation such as one bottle of magnesium citrate is usually sufficient to cleanse the bowels.

After induction of anesthesia, shave the patient and position him or her for surgery. Typically, I shave from nipples to just above the pubic hairline. Place a Foley urethral catheter to drain the bladder and use an orogastric tube to decompress the stomach. After positioning, prep and drape the patient for surgery.

OPERATING ROOM CONFIGURATION AND PATIENT POSITIONING

Anesthesia is located at the head of the table. The surgeon and assistant stand facing the ventral surface of the patient. The scrub nurse and scrub table are situated opposite the operating surgeon and assistant approximately at the level of the patient's waist. Situate a Mayo stand at the level of the patient's upper thigh, and place a monitor opposite the operating surgeon and assistant. Position the insufflation equipment and light source with the monitor facing the surgical team.

The actual position of the surgeon and assistant vary according to the side operated. As a rule of thumb, the assistant operates the camera standing to the left of the surgeon (Fig. 7–1).

The operating room is set up so that the surgeon and assistant can easily view the procedure on the monitors (see Fig. 7–1). Place the patient in the lateral decubitus or flank position. Place the arms on an arm board or in a sling at a 90-degree angle to the surgical table. Place the patient on a beanbag cushion leaned back slightly, about 30 degrees. Carefully pad all pressure points. Bend the bottom leg and place a pillow between the legs for padding. Place a roll in the axilla to prevent brachial plexus injury. Once positioned, suction the air from

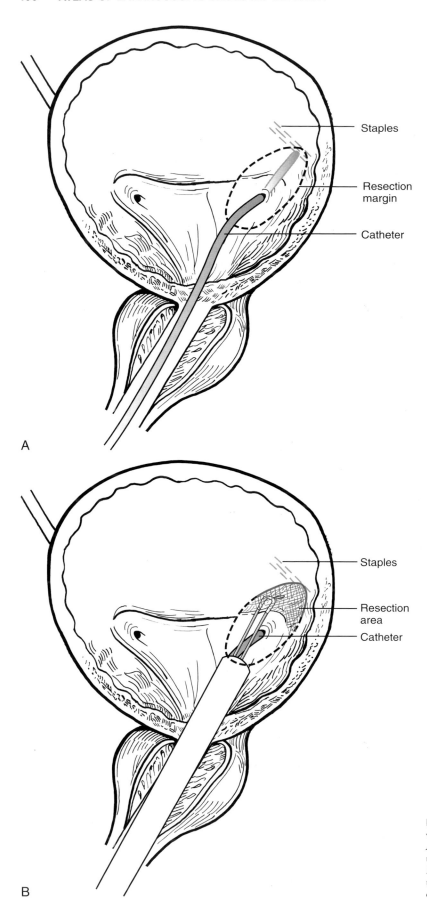

Staples

Resection
margin

Catheter

A

Staples

Resection
area

Catheter

B

FIGURE 8–7. Endoscopic unroofing and fulguration of the intravesical tunnel following extravesical stapling of the bladder cuff. *A*, A whistle-tip catheter is introduced via the cystoscope into the ureteral orifice and advanced to the occluding row of staples. *B*, The Collins electrocautery knife mounted on a 24-French resectoscope is used to incise the intravesical tunnel over the introduced catheter.

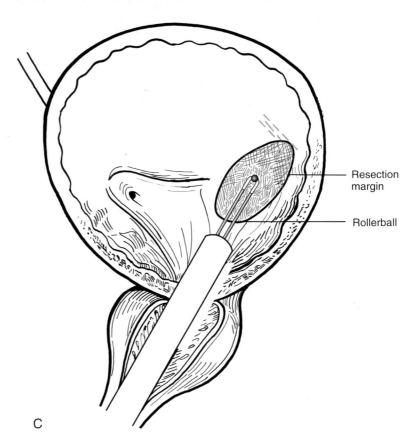

Resection margin

Rollerball

FIGURE 8–7, cont'd. *C,* The whistle-tip catheter has been removed and the rollerball electrode is used to fulgurate the edges and base of the incised intravesical ureter.

C

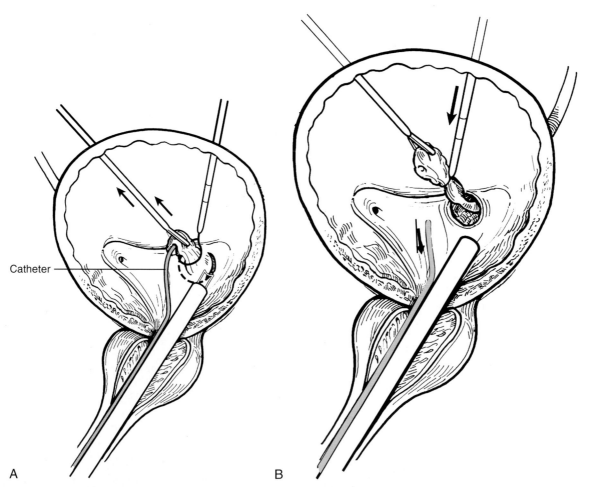

Catheter

A

B

FIGURE 8–8. Transvesical laparoendoscopic management of the distal ureter and associated bladder cuff. *A,* Small transvesical laparoscopic ports are used to position an EndoLoop over the affected ureter through which an open-ended catheter has been inserted. A laparoscopic grasper is used to retract the ureter medially as a Collins knife mounted on a 24-French resectoscope begins incision of the bladder cuff. *B,* The open-ended catheter is withdrawn and the EndoLoop is tightened on the mobilized ureter to prevent efflux of tumor cells.

Endoscopic Release "Pluck"

Perform an initial endoscopic release of the ureter with or without a surrounding cuff of bladder using the Collins knife mounted on a resectoscope. Continue the dissection circumferentially until the perivesical fat is visualized in all areas. Before release, insert a floppy-tipped wire and catheter via the cystoscope into the distal ureter to facilitate the dissection, if needed. Use a 7-French 11.5-mm ureteral occlusion balloon catheter to prevent the efflux of tumor cells as previously described. During the endoscopic portion of the procedure, it is critical to minimize irrigation to reduce the amount of extravasation and the potential for developing a large retroperitoneal collection and resultant hyponatremia.[11] Continue the dissection until the ureter is completely free of all detrusor attachments, then remove the ureteral catheter and insert a 24-French Foley catheter. If an occlusion balloon catheter is used, secure it to the Foley catheter and leave it in place during repositioning.

Then place the patient in a flank position and perform a hand-assisted laparoscopic nephrectomy as previously described. As dissection of the ureter approaches the ureterovesical junction, place gentle cephalad traction on the ureter and divide all small feeding vessels until the ureter is completely free of the bladder and the specimen is removed. Clip the ureter as soon as it is identified to prevent extrusion of tumor cells. If an occlusion balloon catheter is present, clip the ureter directly across the catheter-containing ureter, if needed. Then transect the occlusion catheter as it exits the bladder and deliver its distal segment with the specimen while withdrawing the proximal end from the urethra.

Wong and Leveillee[10] described a similar endoscopic "pluck" technique performed following completion of the hand-assisted laparoscopic nephrectomy that takes advantage of the introduced hand and does not require repositioning. In this approach, place the patient in a modified dorsal lithotomy position with the side of pathology elevated 30 degrees. Support the patient in position using a beanbag and an axillary roll. Secure the legs in low Allen stirrups to provide simultaneous urethral access, and place the ipsilateral arm in an abducted internally rotated position on an arm support. Prep the genitals into the surgical field, and insert a sterile Foley catheter. Then perform a hand-assisted laparoscopic nephrectomy as outlined earlier with early clipping of the ureter to prevent extrusion of tumor cells. After distal dissection of the ureter to the level of the ureterovesical junction, introduce the 24-French resectoscope with the attached Collins knife, and release the ureteral orifice and surrounding bladder cuff as described earlier. Use the introduced hand to gently retract and present the detrusor attachments as the dissection proceeds until the specimen is completely freed and delivered via the hand-assist port. Do not close the bladder defect, reinsert the Foley catheter, and close the ports as outlined later.

Exit the Abdomen and Close the Port Site

Position a 15-French round Davol drain in the ipsilateral pelvis and bring it out through a lateral port site for procedures where the bladder is left open. Close the fascial incision at each of the 10/12-mm port sites using a grasping needle closure device such as the Carter-Thomason (Inlet Medical, Eden Prairie, MN) and a 0 Vicryl suture. Use the introduced hand to assist in transferring the suture from the jaws of the needle grasper after it punctures the fascia.

Perform complete inspection of the dissection site under standard (15 mm Hg) and low (5 mm Hg) insufflation pressures. Use the harmonic shears and electrocautery to obtain hemostasis. Apply a small sheet of surgical cellulose, if needed, to the area of the transected hilar stumps and along the edge of the retained adrenal gland to facilitate hemostasis in these regions. Remove the 5-mm ports, if present, under direct vision, followed by the 10/12-mm trocars, which are withdrawn with the hand protecting the viscera and omentum from becoming entrapped in the closure.

Thoroughly decompress the abdomen, and then position the omentum over the bowel beneath the hand-port incision. Close the peritoneum at this site as a separate layer to prevent subfascial herniations using a running 2-0 chromic suture and use a 1-PDS suture on the fascia. Irrigate the subcutaneous tissues of the hand-assist incision and port sites with antibiotic solution, and reapproximate the skin using a running subcuticular stitch and Steri-Strips. Apply a sterile island or gauze dressing to the hand incision and use Band-Aids or gauze and Tegaderm to cover the port sites.

POSTOPERATIVE MANAGEMENT

Patients are encouraged to begin ambulation on the evening of their surgery. A clear liquid diet is begun once active bowel sounds are present, typically the morning after surgery, and is advanced as tolerated. Pain management consists of intravenous narcotic as needed, which is converted to oral narcotic once bowel function returns. The drain, if present, is continued until outputs average less than 30 mL/8-hour shift on two consecutive shifts. If questions exist regarding a persistent urine leak, the drain fluid can be sent for a creatinine level, which should correspond with serum levels when no leak is present. The drain can be left in place longer if the drain fluid creatinine is elevated. Patients are discharged to home when tolerating a regular diet with adequate pain control on oral medication; typically, this occurs on postoperative day 2 or 3. A Foley catheter is left in place for approximately 7 to 10 days for procedures where the bladder is left open. An office-based cystogram can be performed on the day of planned removal to confirm lack of extravasation. In patients who had the bladder cuff secured using a stapling device, the Foley catheter is removed on the day of discharge. Cancer follow-up including office-based cystoscopy, chest radiographs, and abdominal/pelvic imaging are performed identical to that for patients undergoing open nephroureterectomy.

COMPLICATIONS

In a prospective comparison between hand-assisted laparoscopic and open surgical nephroureterectomy, Seifman and associates[4] reported 19% major and 19% minor complication rates of hand-assisted laparoscopic nephroureterectomy compared with 45% and 27%, respectively, for its open counterpart. Minor complications included ileus, wound infection, and urethral catheter obstruction, and major complications included two patients with respiratory failure requiring reintubation and one death due to cardiac arrhythmia on postoperative day 27. In their series of 22 hand-assisted laparoscopic nephroureterectomies, Stifelman and colleagues[5] reported no intraoperative and only one postoperative complication. This consisted of a patient who developed thrombophlebitis of the right external jugular vein due to intravenous line placement.

Landman and associates[13] compared 16 hand-assisted with 11 standard laparoscopic nephroureterectomies and reported complication rates of 31% and 45%, respectively. A single patient (6%) in the hand-assist group was converted to an open procedure due to failure to progress. Postoperative complications in one patient undergoing hand-assist laparoscopic nephroureterectomy included respiratory failure due to pneumonia with eventual myocardial infarction and sudden death 3 weeks following surgery. Other postoperative complications included two patients with ileus, one of whom also developed a pneumonia, and another patient who required a postoperative transfusion of 2 units of packed red blood cells.

Urinary extravasation has been reported for both hand-assisted and standard laparoscopic surgery and usually can be managed with prolonged catheterization and percutaneous drain placement if necessary.[8,11] Gill and colleagues[11] reported draining the retroperitoneum through a Gibson incision in a patient in whom a transvesical laparoscopic distal ureterectomy with bladder cuff excision was performed first followed by a standard laparoscopic nephroureterectomy. This patient also had the resultant complication of fluid absorption and hyponatremia.

Pelvic and retroperitoneal tumor seeding have been reported for open and laparoscopic nephroureterectomy and is thought to be an increased risk when an initial endoscopic "pluck" technique is used.[8] High tumor grade and stage were the common features of three cases of retroperitoneal tumor recurrence following laparoscopic nephroureterectomy in the series from Washington University.[8]

SUMMARY

The hand-assist device can serve as a useful adjunct when performing a laparoscopic nephroureterectomy. A number of techniques are available for managing the distal ureter, and, in part, the approach is determined by the grade and location of the patient's cancer in addition to the surgeon's preference.

Tips and Tricks

- Insertion of instruments directly through the matrix of the GelPort hand-assist device often obviates the need for insertion of an additional port when performing the distal ureteral dissection.
- It is almost always necessary to transect the superior vesical artery to gain adequate entrance into the intravesical tunnel when the Endo-GIA stapler is going to be applied to the ureter and attached bladder cuff.
- An open-ended, whistle-tip, or dilating balloon catheter can be inserted into the intravesical tunnel to facilitate endoscopic unroofing. It is not necessary to use an occluding balloon if the nephrectomy portion of the operation is performed first and a clip is placed on the proximal ureter.
- Irrigation should be kept to a minimum when performing an initial endoscopic release of the bladder cuff and distal ureter to prevent significant retroperitoneal extravasation and absorption.

REFERENCES

1. Clayman RV, Kavoussi LR, Fienshau RS, et al: Laparoscopic nephroureterectomy: Initial clinical case report. J Laparoendosc Surg 1:343–349, 1991.
2. Nakada SY, Moon TD, Gist M, et al: Use of the pneumo sleeve as an adjunct in laparoscopic nephrectomy. Urology 49:612–613, 1997.
3. Wolf JF Jr, Moon TD, Nakada SY: Hand assisted laparoscopic nephrectomy, comparison to standard laparoscopic nephrectomy. J Urol 160:22–27, 1998.
4. Seifman BD, Montie JE, Wolf JS Jr: Prospective comparison between hand assisted laparoscopic and open surgical nephroureterectomy for urothelial cell carcinoma. Urology 57:133–137, 2001.
5. Stifelman MD, Sosa RE, Andrade A, et al: Hand-assisted nephroureterectomy for the treatment of transitional cell carcinoma of the upper urinary tract. Urology 56:741–747, 2000.
6. Cannon GM Jr, Averch T, Colen J, et al: Hand-assisted laparoscopic nephroureterectomy with open cystotomy for removal of the distal ureter and bladder cuff. J Endourol 19:973–975, 2005.
7. Chen J, Shih-Chieh C, Wen-Tsong H, et al: Modified approach of hand-assisted laparoscopic nephroureterectomy for transitional cell carcinoma of the upper urinary tract. Urology 58:930–934, 2001.
8. Shalhav AL, Dunn MD, Portis AJ, et al: Laparoscopic nephroureterectomy for upper transitional cell cancer: The Washington University experience. J Urol 163:1100–1104, 2000.
9. Gonzalez CM, Batler RA, Schoor RA, et al: A novel endoscopic approach towards resection of the distal ureter with surrounding bladder cuff during hand assisted laparoscopic nephroureterectomy. J Urol 165:483–485, 2001.
10. Wong C, Leveillee RJ: Hand-assisted laparoscopic nephroureterectomy with cystoscopic en bloc excision of the distal ureter and bladder cuff. J Endourol 16:329–333, 2002.
11. Gill IS, Soble JJ, Miller SD, et al: A novel technique for management of the en bloc bladder cuff and distal ureter during laparoscopic nephroureterectomy. J Urol 161:430–434, 1999.
12. Lee DI, Landman J: Novel approach to minimizing trocar sites during challenging hand-assisted laparoscopic surgery utilizing the Gelport: Trans-gel instrument insertion and utilization. J Endourol 17:69–71, 2003.
13. Landman J, Lev RY, Bhayani S, et al: Comparison of hand assisted and standard laparoscopic radical nephroureterectomy for the management of localized transitional cell carcinoma. J Urol 167:2387–2391, 2002.

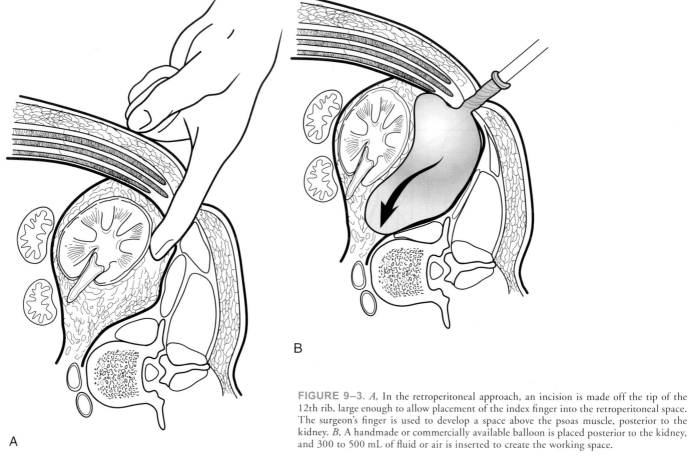

FIGURE 9–3. *A,* In the retroperitoneal approach, an incision is made off the tip of the 12th rib, large enough to allow placement of the index finger into the retroperitoneal space. The surgeon's finger is used to develop a space above the psoas muscle, posterior to the kidney. *B,* A handmade or commercially available balloon is placed posterior to the kidney, and 300 to 500 mL of fluid or air is inserted to create the working space.

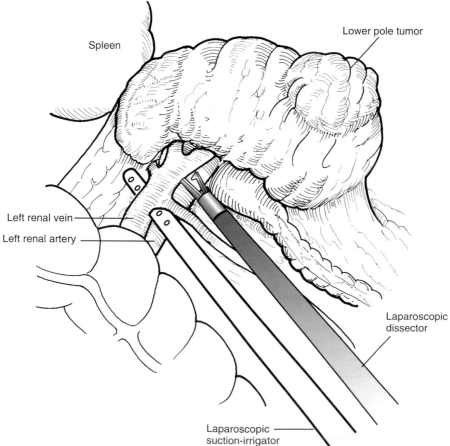

FIGURE 9–4. Careful dissection of the renal artery and renal vein allows complete occlusion and hilar control of the blood vessels to create a bloodless field for dissection of the renal mass.

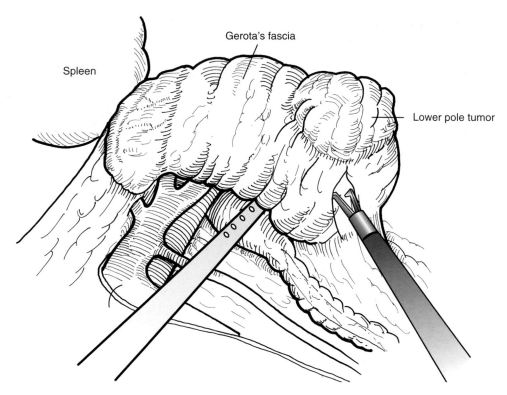

FIGURE 9–5. Gerota's fascia is opened near the renal mass, and the surface of the uninvolved kidney is identified.

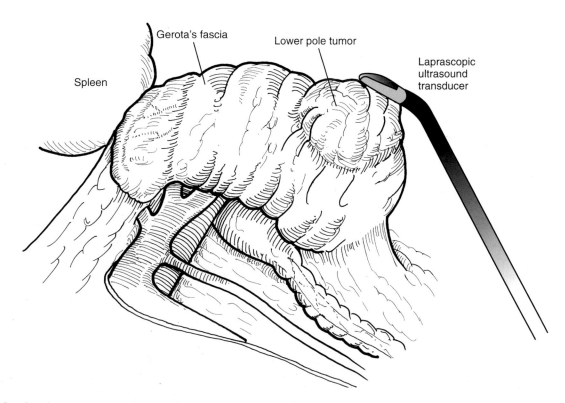

FIGURE 9–6. When the tumor is not readily identified with visual inspection or is endophytic, laparoscopic ultrasound is used to locate the mass.

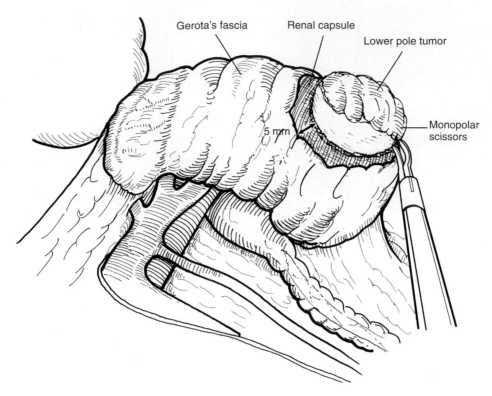

FIGURE 9–7. Electrocautery from closed monopolar scissors is used to score renal parenchyma at least 5 mm from tumor to delineate intended line of dissection.

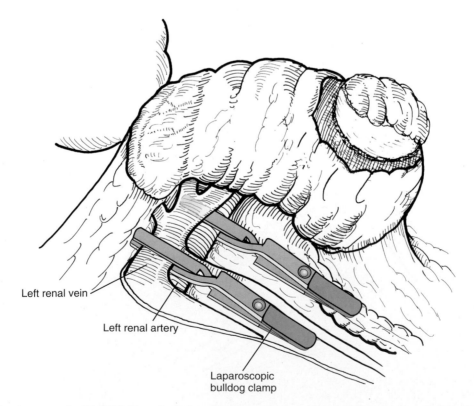

FIGURE 9–8. Vascular clamps are placed individually on both the renal artery and vein, or the renal hilum can be occluded with a vascular clamp inserted through a separate trocar site.

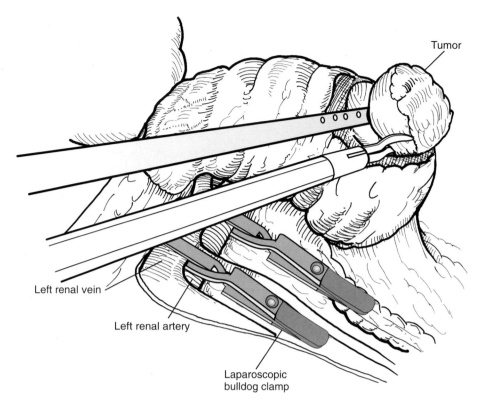

FIGURE 9–9. The irrigator-aspirator tip is used for countertraction and to maintain a bloodless field while cold scissors are used to excise lesion.

ning of the case. If a collecting system violation is noted, oversew it with interrupted 3-0 Vicryl sutures (Fig. 9–10).

Oversew cut arteries or veins that are identified in the renal defect with 3-0 Vicryl sutures. Then fill the renal parenchymal defect with a single or combination of hemostatic agents (FloSeal or Tisseel [Baxter Healthcare Corp., Deerfield, IL], Surgicel [Johnson & Johnson, New Brunswick, NJ], gelfoam and thrombin, and so on) (Fig. 9–11). If Surgicel bolsters are used, place 3-0 Vicryl sutures anchored to the adjacent renal parenchyma across the bolsters to secure them in place and to compress the edges of the renal defect (Fig. 9–12).

Release the vascular clamp and observe the renal defect for hemorrhage. Compression with a mini-lap pad placed through the 12-mm port before hilar clamping may help establish hemostasis. Decrease the pneumoperitoneum to less than 10 mm Hg for 5 to 10 minutes while continuously observing for bleeding. Once adequate hemostasis has been ensured, place a closed suction drain in the paracolic gutter adjacent to the kidney but not overlying the renal defect.

Use a Carter-Thomason closure device with a 0 Vicryl suture to close the 10/12-mm trocar sites under direct laparoscopic vision, ensuring that no vital structures are entrapped. Release CO_2 from the abdomen, and close the skin incisions in a running subcuticular fashion.

Retroperitoneal Approach

Make a 15-mm incision in the area of Petit's triangle, just below the tip of the 12th rib, and extend the dissection downward through the lumbodorsal fascia and into the retroperitoneal space with the aid of a clamp. Bluntly dissect this space with the tip of a finger along the psoas muscle posterior to the kidney. Next,

place a balloon dilator through this tract, and, under vision, further expand the retroperitoneal space. Introduce a 10-mm camera via this trocar, and establish a pneumoretroperitoneum of 15 mm Hg. Expand and cinch the trocar cuff to the skin to prevent CO_2 leakage. View pertinent structures for orientation and to exclude entry trauma: the psoas muscle with overlying intact fascia and ureter, inferiorly; intact Gerota's fascia surrounding the kidney, cephalad; and intact peritoneal membrane, anteriorly. Place the other trocars as described previously, and further expand the retroperitoneal space by bluntly sweeping the peritoneum anteriorly (see Fig. 9–3).

Retract the kidney upward and cephalad while bluntly dissecting it off the psoas fascia. The pulsation of the renal artery is then evident and guides the approach to its dissection. Dissect the renal artery and vein to the point of allowing easy placement of bulldog clamps when needed. Next, use intraoperative US to verify the location and extent of the renal lesion. Enter Gerota's fascia away from the area of the lesion, and remove the lesion as described for the intraperitoneal approach after clamping the vessels.

With either laparoscopic approach, minimize warm ischemia time (<30 minutes, not >1 hour) because clamp times within this time period have been shown not to result in long-term renal dysfunction.[8]

POSTOPERATIVE MANAGEMENT

Important immediate postoperative considerations include, but are not limited to, monitoring of vital signs and quantity and content of drain output. Delayed bleeding may occur for up to 30 days after partial nephrectomy[9]; therefore, it is imperative

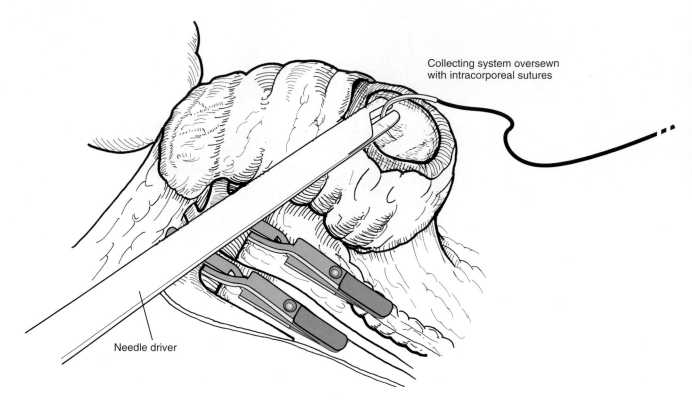

Collecting system oversewn
with intracorporeal sutures

Needle driver

FIGURE 9–10. Entry into the collecting system is common and can usually be seen without assistance. Some surgeons place an open-ended catheter at the beginning of the case and use retrograde injection of methylene blue to identify sites where the collecting system has been transected. Collecting system injury is repaired with 3-0 absorbable suture. The Lapra-Ty clip (Ethicon Endo-Surgery, Cincinnati, OH) can be placed on the end of the suture as a knot, and a second clip is applied to secure the suture.

to keep in mind that bleeding remains at the forefront of potential complications. Continued renal hemorrhage may manifest itself as persistent or copious bloody drain output, hematuria, or unstable vital signs.

We recommend early ambulation to minimize the risk of deep venous thrombosis; however, 24 hours of postoperative bedrest is routinely prescribed by others.[9] Furthermore, we restrict strenuous exercise for at least 1 month to allow adequate healing of the partial nephrectomy bed.

If an orogastric tube or a ureteral catheter has been placed, remove it immediately postoperatively. Allow the Foley catheter to remain overnight. Note drain output volume and whether it increases after Foley catheter removal because this may be an indication of vesicoureteral reflux into a persistent or unrecognized renal collecting system injury.

Monitoring the drain fluid creatinine concentration may help differentiate peritoneal fluid from urine and assist in deciding on drain removal. Remove the drain only when the fluid content is consistent with peritoneal fluid, in color and chemical composition.

COMPLICATIONS

Complications following laparoscopic partial nephrectomy can generally be divided into intraoperative and postoperative categories. The most common intraoperative complication that can be attributed directly to the laparoscopic nature of this technique is hemorrhage, occurring in 3.5% in one of the largest published series.[9] Intraoperative hemorrhage is invariably due to inadequate vascular control technique. Some have

found that laparoscopic bulldog clamps, which are often used for the retroperitoneoscopic approach, provide suboptimal vascular occlusion compared with Satinsky clamps. We have not found this to be true, and Satinsky clamps are not infallible. In addition to clamp failure, failure to identify and control multiple renal arteries also may result in intraoperative hemorrhage. If the hemorrhage cannot be controlled quickly, conversion to open surgery is indicated.

Postoperative complications directly attributable to the laparoscopic technique are also typically related to hemorrhage or renal collecting system injury. Postoperative or delayed unprovoked spontaneous hemorrhage from the partial nephrectomy bed has been described as occurring up to 14 days postoperatively and in 6% of patients.[9] Bedrest with spontaneous resolution, segmental arterial embolization, or completion nephrectomy are the usual treatment measures, depending on the severity of hemorrhage.

Renal collecting system injury also occurs intraoperatively,[9] sometimes from necessity to completely excise a large or more centrally located lesion. Such injuries may not be recognized immediately. Aforementioned techniques to identify such injuries are available. Most surgeons recommend immediate closure of large defects, but opinions differ on the need to close smaller ones.

Significant renal collecting system leaks usually manifest perioperatively as persistent drain output consistent with urine. Delayed presentation of unrecognized leaks usually manifests as urinomas, symptomatic or asymptomatic. Management in the perioperative period may consist of collecting system decompression via ipsilateral ureteral stenting and/or Foley catheter replacement or simple prolongation of the drainage

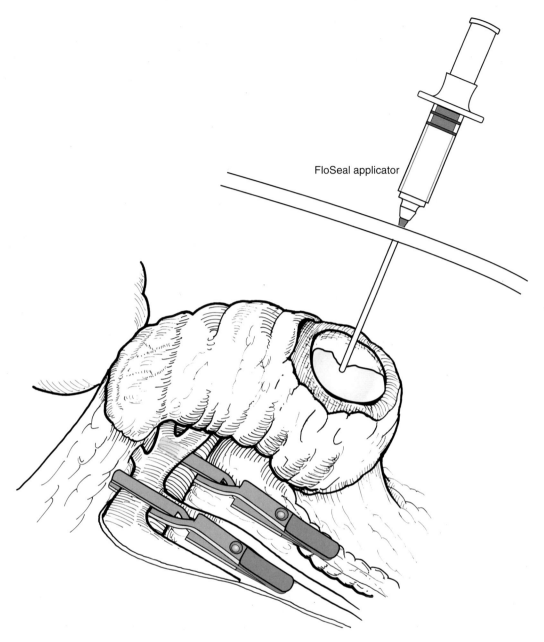

FloSeal applicator

FIGURE 9–11. Hemostatic and sealing fibrin product is applied to the surface of the kidney using a laparoscopic applicator through a trocar near the kidney.

period. Urinomas may be managed by percutaneous drainage, by observation with ureteral stenting, or by observation alone, depending on size and symptomatology.

Other less commonly occurring serious complications include ureteral injury, renal dysfunction, and vascular injuries.

SUMMARY

Technological advances have allowed complex laparoscopic surgery to be performed by urologic surgeons. Laparoscopic partial nephrectomy, which combines both extirpation and renal reconstruction, emulates the open surgical procedure. This is true for both the transperitoneal and retroperitoneal approach. As our field tries to improve the care we provide for patients with renal masses, laparoscopic partial nephrectomy offers these patients a sound oncologic treatment that causes less pain and suffering than is associated with open renal surgery.

Tips and Tricks

- For obese patients, it is often helpful to shift all trocar positions laterally to place them closer to the kidney. This often obviates the need for extra-long instrumentation and for placing undue torque on the trocars with upward retraction. Care should be taken to avoid injuring the epigastric vessels.
- Grasping Gerota's fascia with a Debakey forceps and providing careful upward retraction of the kidney often facilitate hilar identification and dissection.
- Use of Lapra-Ty clips (Ethicon Endo-Surgery, Cincinnati, OH) on each end of sutures decreases warm ischemia time by obviating need for laparoscopic suturing.

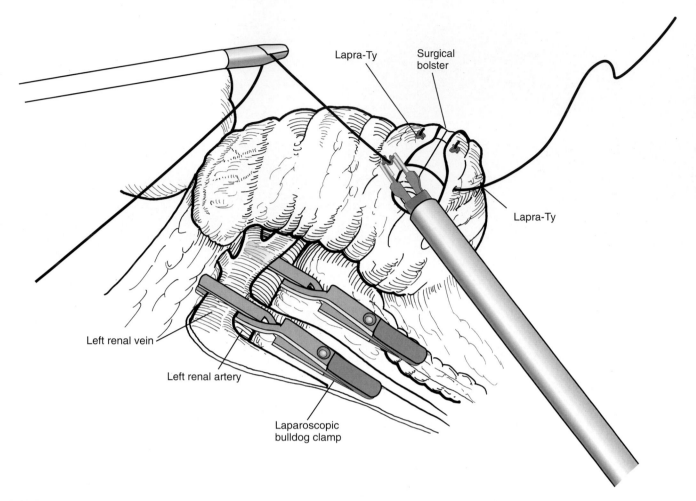

FIGURE 9–12. Hemostatic bolster can be formed by rolling Surgicel, tying each end with an absorbable suture, and placing it in the kidney defect. For large resections, two or more of these bolsters may be necessary. The kidney defect is then approximated with absorbable suture passed approximately 1 cm from the edge of the renal capsule. Lapra-Ty clips can be used to secure both ends of the suture. However, the surgeon must guard against excessive tension on the suture, which can cause the Lapra-Ty to pull through the renal capsule into the kidney.

REFERENCES

1. Chow WH, Devesa SS, Warren JL, et al: Rising incidence of renal cell cancer in the United States. JAMA 281:1628–1631, 1999.
2. Fergany AF, Hafez KS, NoVick AC: Long-term results of nephron sparing surgery for localized renal cell carcinoma: 10-Year followup. J Urol 163:442–445, 2000.
3. Allaf ME, Bhayani SB, Rogers C, et al: Laparoscopic partial nephrectomy: Evaluation of long-term oncological outcome. J Urol 172:871–873, 2004.
4. Winfield HN, Donovan JF, Godet AS, Clayman RV: Laparoscopic partial nephrectomy: Initial case report for benign disease. J Endourol 7:521–526, 1993.
5. Hafez KS, Fergany AF, NoVick AC: Nephron sparing surgery for localized renal cell carcinoma: Impact of tumor size on patient survival, tumor recurrence and TNM staging. J Urol 162:1930–1933, 1999.
6. Finelli A, Gill IS: Laparoscopic partial nephrectomy: Contemporary technique and results. Urol Oncol 22:139–144, 2004.
7. Johnston WK 3rd, Wolf JS Jr: Laparoscopic partial nephrectomy: Technique, oncologic efficacy, and safety. Curr Urol Rep 6:19–28, 2005.
8. Bhayani SB, Rha KH, Pinto PA, et al: Laparoscopic partial nephrectomy: Effect of warm ischemia on serum creatinine. J Urol 172:1264–1266, 2004.
9. Ramani AP, Desai MM, Steinberg AP, et al: Complications of laparoscopic partial nephrectomy in 200 cases. J Urol 173:42–47, 2005.

CHAPTER 10

Laparoscopic Nephroureterectomy

C. William Schwab II
Thomas W. Jarrett

Transitional cell carcinoma of the upper urinary tract comprises 5% of all urothelial tumors and 5% to 10% of renal tumors. Such tumors have a propensity for ipsilateral recurrence and are classically managed with the surgical removal of the ipsilateral kidney, ureter, and surrounding bladder cuff.[1] The standard open nephroureterectomy is performed through a single large incision or two separate incisions and is associated with significant morbidity and a substantial period of convalescence.

In an effort to reduce the invasiveness of the procedure, the technology and innovation of laparoscopic nephrectomy were translated to laparoscopic nephroureterectomy, first performed at Washington University in 1991.[2] Studies have demonstrated this procedure to have reduced morbidity while providing equivalent oncologic control.[3–6] There have been debates over the various approaches: transperitoneal, retroperitoneal, and hand-assisted. No single approach has shown an advantage, and all show decreased morbidity compared with the open counterpart. The approach chosen depends largely on patient factors and surgeon experience.

Controversy continues regarding the optimal approach to and management of the distal ureter and surrounding bladder cuff. The ideal technique would allow reproducible oncologic control paralleling that of open surgery with a minimum degree of invasiveness, complexity, and required operative time. Several techniques have been described using a variety of endoscopic, laparoscopic, and open approaches. Larger series with intermediate and long-term follow-up are beginning to demonstrate differences in local and retroperitoneal recurrence rates between the various techniques.[5–10]

This chapter describes the transperitoneal approach and several accepted surgical techniques for the distal ureter, including the following:

1. Open dissection and excision of distal ureter and bladder cuff
2. Transvesical laparoscopic technique
3. Modified pluck technique
4. Ureteral unroofing technique

INDICATIONS AND CONTRAINDICATIONS

The indications for laparoscopic-assisted nephroureterectomy remain the same as those for open nephroureterectomy. Transitional cell carcinoma of the renal collecting system or ureter is the most commonly encountered indication. Occasionally, benign conditions or nonfunctioning kidneys warrant removal of the entire ipsilateral upper urinary tract.

The only absolute contraindication to laparoscopic-assisted nephroureterectomy is an uncorrected bleeding diathesis. Relative contraindications include situations that may be more challenging for the inexperienced laparoscopist, including the presence of concomitant inflammatory conditions such as tuberculosis or xanthogranulomatous pyelonephritis and patients with a history of ipsilateral renal surgery or extensive intraperitoneal surgery.

Consider kidney-sparing surgery for patients with low-grade, low-stage disease at risk of renal failure following removal of a renal unit, with a single kidney, with bilateral disease, and with Balkan nephropathy.

PATIENT PREOPERATIVE EVALUATION AND PREPARATION

Preoperatively establish the diagnosis of transitional cell carcinoma of the upper tracts in a manner similar to that for open surgery (Fig. 10–1). Confirm upper tract abnormalities or filling defects with ipsilateral cytologic or ureteroscopic evaluation with direct biopsy or localized cytology at the lesions. Completely evaluate to identify the presence of multiple or bilateral tumors.

Staging evaluation includes radiographic evaluation of the chest and cross-sectional imaging of the abdomen and pelvis. Obtain standard laboratory serum studies, including liver function tests. Perform a postoperative nephrologic evaluation on patients with limited renal reserve if postoperative renal failure ensues.

Obtain a preoperative urine culture and, if positive, treat it appropriately. Patients maintain a clear liquid diet for 24 hours preoperatively, and they may do a mild mechanical bowel prep the night of surgery. Blood typing and cross-matching and preoperative antibiotic prophylaxis are routine.

OPERATING ROOM CONFIGURATION AND PATIENT POSITIONING

Laparoscopic-assisted nephroureterectomy has two broad objectives. Dissect and isolate the kidney and ureter distal to the pelvis, then remove an intact specimen for exact pathologic staging (dissection of the distal ureter and bladder cuff is one way to do this). Proper positioning optimizes both portions of the procedure, regardless of the technique chosen to manage the distal cuff because intraoperative repositioning without repeat prepping is feasible.

A modified flank/torque position allows intraoperative repositioning of the patient from a flank position, for the

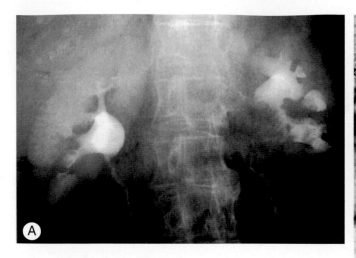

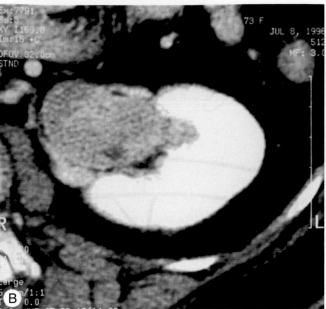

FIGURE 10–1. *A,* Intravenous pyelogram showing large filling defect in the left renal pelvis. *B,* Computed tomography scan confirms mass in the left renal pelvis

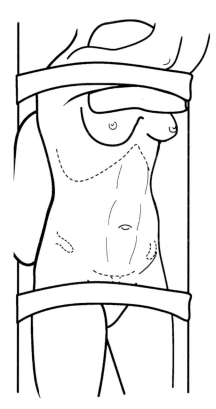

FIGURE 10–2. For laparoscopic nephroureterectomy, the patient is placed in the supine position with the ipsilateral arm across the chest. The patient is secured to the table and may be rotated during the case to the contralateral side.

nephrectomy portion, to a supine position, for the distal ureterectomy portion, without repeat prepping. Bump up the ipsilateral hip, flank, and shoulder to approximately 20 degrees and bring the ipsilateral arm across the table and either place it on a padded arm board or flex it in front of the patient's face on a pillow (Fig. 10–2). An axillary roll is not necessary, but care-

fully pad pressure points. Carefully fix the patient to the bed with wide cloth tape at the shoulders, hips, and lower extremities. Do not flex the table and do not use the kidney bridge. Rotate the bed to ensure the patient's immobility during the procedure. Widely prep the patient and drape to include the flank and the urethra. Place a Foley catheter on the field before beginning. If the procedure starts with the laparoscopic dissection of the kidney and ureter, stand with the assistant on the side contralateral to the tumor (Fig. 10–3).

TROCAR PLACEMENT

Generally, use a transperitoneal, three-port approach; add a fourth port if retraction of liver, spleen, colon, and kidney become necessary. Trocar position depends mainly on the patient's body habitus (Fig. 10–4). Insufflate the abdomen following Veress needle placement in the umbilicus. For patients with prior midline abdominal surgery, shift needle placement lateral to the rectus at the level of the umbilicus. Place a 10/12-mm trocar with a visual obturator through the umbilicus, into the abdomen, under direct vision. Place a second 10/12-mm trocar at the level of the umbilicus just lateral to the rectus muscle. Place a 5-mm trocar in the midline between the umbilicus and the xiphoid process.

For obese patients, placement in the modified flank position creates a disproportionate shift in the pannus such that trocars placed at the umbilicus will actually enter the peritoneum below the midline and farther away from the retroperitoneum. A shift in trocar placement, lateral to the rectus abdominis, allows for improved visualization and working distances.[11]

During the nephrectomy portion of the procedure, situate the camera in the umbilical port and operate through the superior midline and lateral trocar sites. As the dissection continues, place additional 2- or 5-mm trocars as necessary to aid in retraction or dissection. Use a midline port placed just cephalad to the upper port to retract the gallbladder and liver for right-sided lesions. Use a port in the anterior axillary line or lower midline to aid with lateral retraction of the colon (Fig. 10–5).

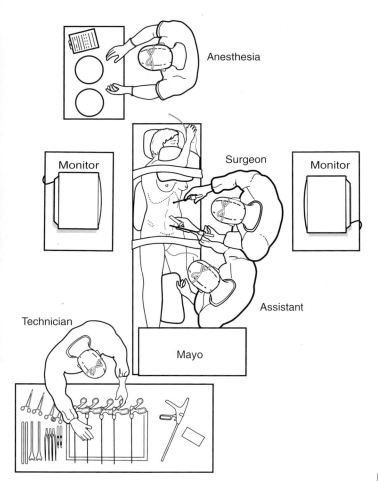

FIGURE 10–3. The surgeon and assistant stand on the contralateral side of the table with the scrub person at the foot of the table.

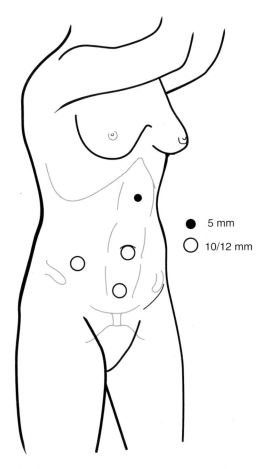

5 mm
10/12 mm

FIGURE 10–4. The trocars are placed in the midline for most patients. Markedly obese patients require a shift of the trocars laterally to allow for adequate visualization of the renal hilum and pelvic structures.

Alternatively, pass a suture on a straight needle through the abdominal wall and under the structure to be elevated or retracted, and pass the needle back out through the anterior abdominal wall. Then fix the suture in place with a hemostat (see Fig. 10–7). A low midline port can be helpful for dissection of the distal ureter.

PROCEDURE

Colon Mobilization

Following trocar placement, rotate the table to place the patient in a flank position. Incise the posterior peritoneum at the line of Toldt, allowing mobilization and displacement of the colon mesentery medial to the aorta on the right and vena cava on the left. For a right-sided dissection, carry the incision from the iliac vessels to the hepatic flexure. For a left-sided dissection, carry the incision cephalad to the splenic flexure (Fig. 10–6). Obtain retraction assistance using a straight needle passed from outside directly into the abdomen, around the ureter, and then back outside the abdomen (Fig. 10–7). Divide the renocolic ligaments to allow further mobilization of the colon off the lower pole of the kidney. Leave the lateral attachments of Gerota's fascia to prevent the kidney from falling medially during the dissection of the hilum (Fig. 10–8).

Nephrectomy

Identify the ureter medial to the lower pole of the kidney and dissect the ureter toward the renal hilum. Maintain a wide margin of tissue if an invasive ureteral tumor is known or suspected (Fig. 10–9). Carry the dissection cephalad to the renal hilum. Then carefully dissect and identify the major vessels. Ligate and divide the renal artery either with an endovascular gastrointestinal anastomosis device (GIA) or with multiple 10-mm clips and Endo Shears (Fig. 10–10). Apply a similar technique to any accessory arteries.

Next, turn attention to the renal vein. Identify lumbar, adrenal, and accessory veins and divide them between clips. Divide the renal vein with an endovascular GIA or locking clips (Fig. 10–11). Fully mobilize the kidney either inside or outside Gerota's fascia, depending on the tumor location and stage. Dissect with electrocautery or a harmonic scalpel to maintain hemostasis while freeing the upper pole of attachments (Fig. 10–12).

Distal Ureteral Dissection

Clip the ureter to prevent distal migration of tumor cells in the subsequent portion of the procedure. Continue the peritoneal incision in the inferior direction over the iliac vessels and medial to the median umbilical ligament to completely expose the ureter (Fig. 10–13). Carry out ureteral dissection as far distally

Text continued on page 128

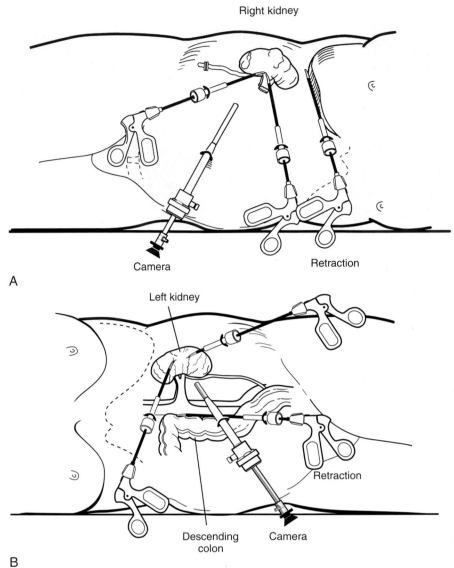

Right kidney

Camera

Retraction

A

Left kidney

Retraction

Descending
colon

Camera

B

FIGURE 10–5. Accessory ports are placed as needed to retract surrounding organs. *A,* For right-sided lesions, a port below the xiphoid is helpful for retracting the liver. *B,* On the left side, a lower midline port is helpful for retracting the descending colon.

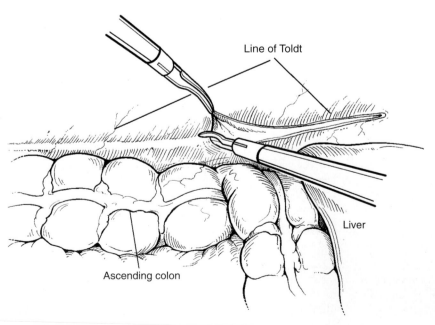

Line of Toldt

Liver

Ascending colon

FIGURE 10–6. The lateral attachments of the colon are divided along the white line of Toldt followed by the reno-colic attachments. The colon mesentery is mobilized medial to the aorta.

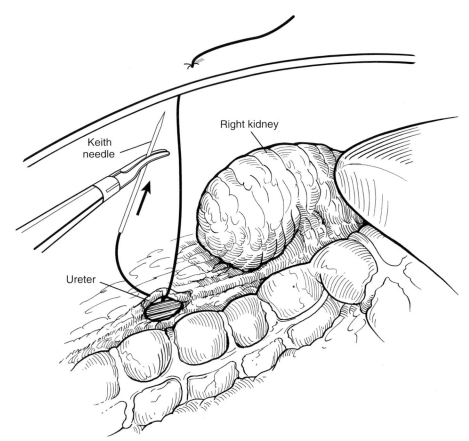

FIGURE 10–7. A suture on a straight needle can be used to elevate the ureter and assist with dissection.

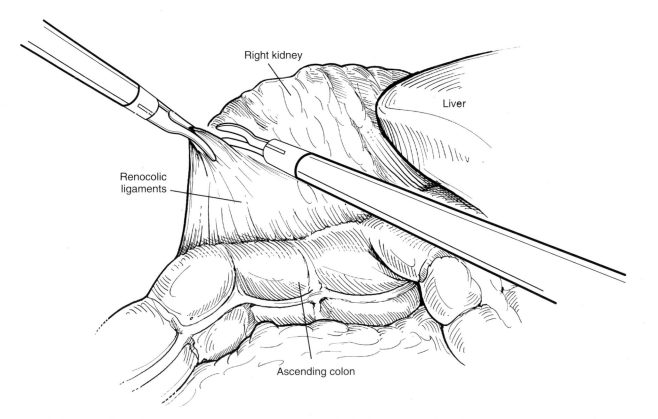

FIGURE 10–8. The renocolic attachments are freed from the kidney to expose the duodenum and renal vessels.

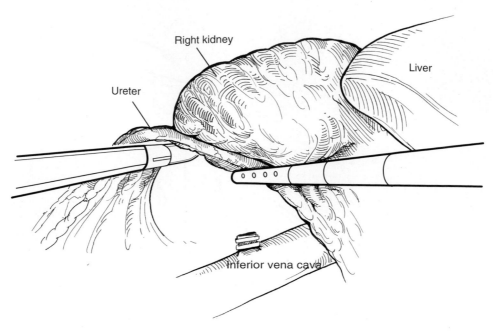

FIGURE 10–9. Once the bowel is reflected medially, a grasper is placed under the lower pole of the kidney placing the renal vessels on stretch. The renal hilum can then safely be dissected.

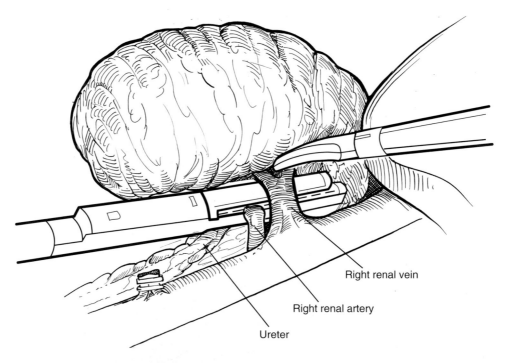

FIGURE 10–10. The renal artery is divided with an endovascular stapler.

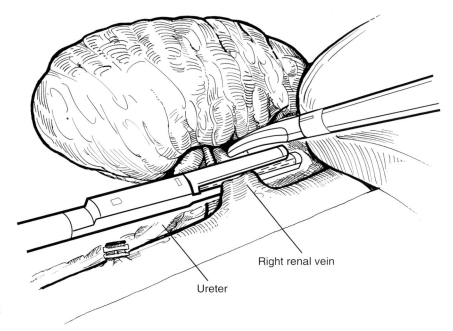

Right renal vein

Ureter

FIGURE 10–11. The renal vein is divided after the renal artery using the endoscopic vascular stapling device.

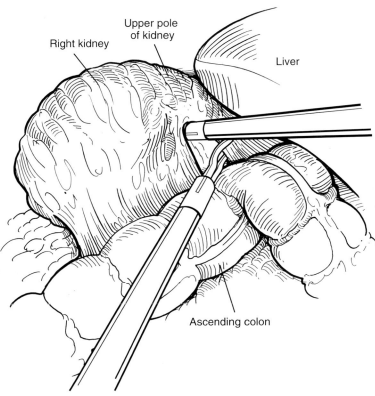

Right kidney

Upper pole of kidney

Liver

Ascending colon

FIGURE 10–12. The upper pole attachments are divided, freeing the entire kidney.

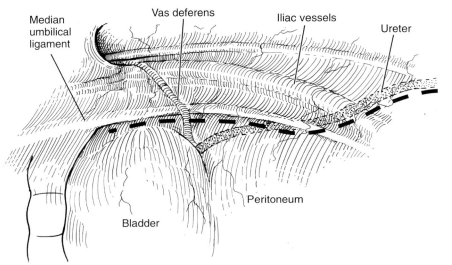

Median umbilical ligament

Vas deferens

Iliac vessels

Ureter

Peritoneum

Bladder

FIGURE 10–13. The peritoneal incision is extended deep into the pelvis over the iliac vessels and medial to the median umbilical ligament.

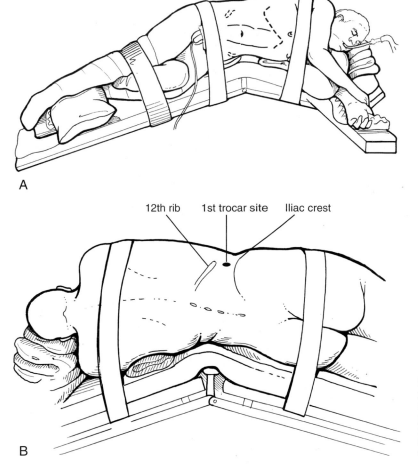

12th rib   1st trocar site   Iliac crest

FIGURE 12–4. *A,* For a retroperitoneal approach, the patient is placed in the full flank position with the lower leg flexed and the upper leg straight. An axillary roll is used, and the lower arm is placed on an arm board. The upper arm can be flexed across a pillow or placed on an elevated arm support. *B,* The kidney rest is elevated and the table is flexed. The patient is secured to the table with padded straps along the hips and upper extremities.

Retroperitoneal Approach

Typically, use three trocars for a retroperitoneal approach. The first is a 10/12-mm trocar placed in the posterior axillary line halfway between the iliac crest and the tip of the 12th rib (Fig. 12–6). After dissecting a space in the retroperitoneum and sweeping the peritoneum medially, place the second 10/12-mm trocar in the anterior axillary line under direct vision. Place a third, 5-mm, trocar superiorly, above the 10/12-mm trocar in the anterior axillary line. Avoid placing this trocar in a supracostal location because this may lead to inadvertent entry into the pleural space.

PROCEDURE

Transperitoneal Approach

After trocar placement, rotate the patient maximally toward the surgeon. On the left side, reflect the descending colon medially from the splenic flexure to the level of the sigmoid entering the pelvis. At the level of the spleen, divide the phrenocolic, lienorenal, and splenocolic ligaments (Fig. 12–7). On the right side, reflect the colon along the line of Toldt to the cecum (Fig. 12–8). Perform this with sharp and blunt dissection using

electrocautery as necessary. It may be necessary to use an instrument to facilitate liver retraction. Divide the colorenal ligaments. Be cautious not to injure the duodenum during division of the medial attachments. For interpolar or medial lesions, perform a Kocher maneuver to provide excellent exposure (Fig. 12–9). Do this with a combination of sharp and blunt dissection while avoiding cautery in the vicinity of the duodenum. If the correct planes are dissected, there is minimal bleeding.

Once the colorenal ligaments have been divided, Gerota's fascia can be seen. Often, the renal cyst is easily seen at this point and looks like a well-defined blue dome protruding from the surface of the kidney (Fig. 12–10). If it is difficult to identify the cyst location or if there is concern that the mass is not a simple cyst, perform intraoperative ultrasonography (US) using a laparoscopic probe to locate and further characterize the lesion. After visual inspection, aspirate the cyst through the 5-mm port using a laparoscopic needle (Fig. 12–11), and send the fluid for cytologic and chemical analysis.

After aspiration, excise the cyst wall with laparoscopic scissors at its junction with the parenchyma and send it for pathologic evaluation (Fig. 12–12). Due to the possibility of malignancy, remove the specimen via a laparoscopic bag device. It is also possible to send the cyst wall for frozen section. Obtain biopsy samples from the base of the cyst using the 5-mm laparoscopic biopsy forceps (Fig. 12–13). Fulgurate the base of the

Text continued on page 151

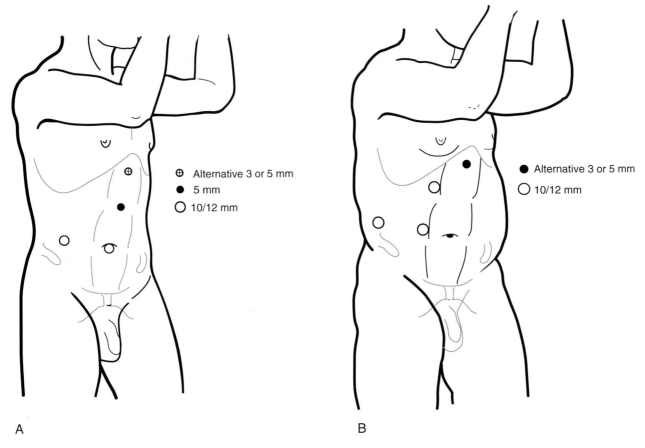

FIGURE 12–5. *A,* In a transabdominal approach, three trocars are used. The first 10/12-mm port is placed lateral to the rectus muscle at the level of the umbilicus. A second 10/12-mm port is placed at the umbilicus, and this is used for the 30-degree lens. The third port is a 5-mm port placed in the midline halfway between the umbilicus and xyphoid. *B,* In obese patients, the ports are shifted laterally.

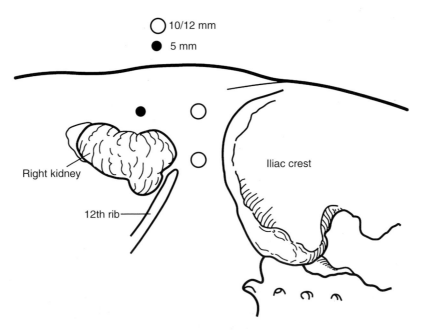

FIGURE 12–6. Typical port placement for the retroperitoneal approach.

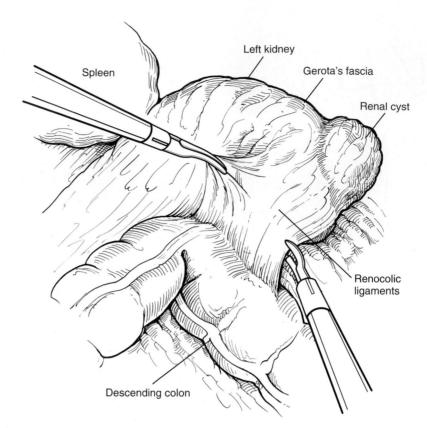

FIGURE 12–7. Division of the phrenocolic, lienorenal, and splenocolic ligaments on a left-sided dissection.

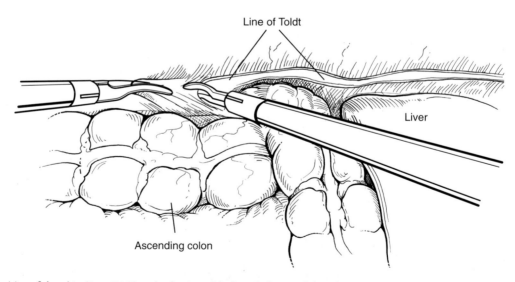

FIGURE 12–8. Incision of the white line of Toldt and reflection of the hepatic flexure of the colon.

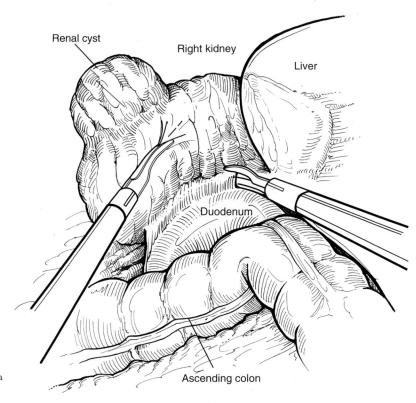

FIGURE 12–9. On the right side, the colon is reflected and a Kocher maneuver may be necessary to expose the kidney.

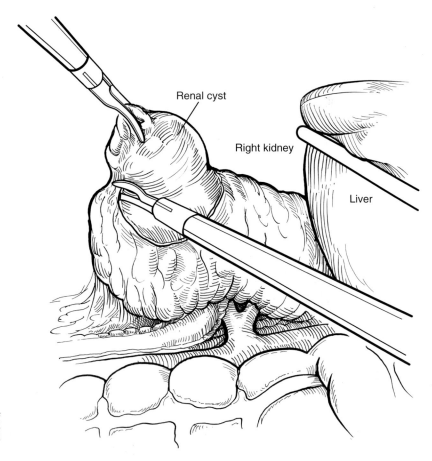

FIGURE 12–10. The cyst is located after reflecting the bowel and incising Gerota's fascia. A laparoscopic ultrasound probe may be needed to locate small or intraparenchymal cysts.

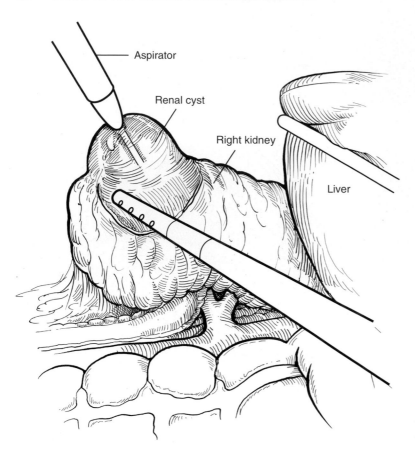

Aspirator

Renal cyst

Right kidney

Liver

FIGURE 12–11. After visual inspection, the cyst is aspirated through the 5-mm port by means of a laparoscopic cyst aspiration needle (aspirator).

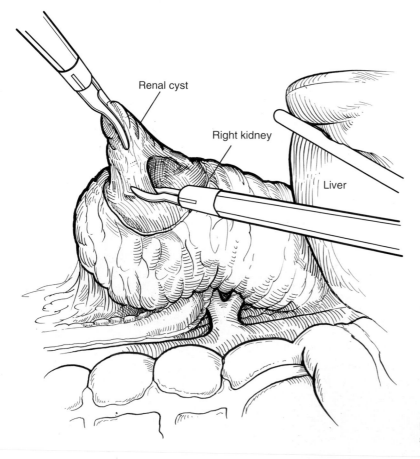

Renal cyst

Right kidney

Liver

FIGURE 12–12. The cyst wall is elevated with a grasper, and scissors are used to circumferentially excise the cyst wall.

Lapa
Perc
of R
Tech

Technologic ad
lutionizing the
nephrectomy is
it has been show
recently, initial
nephrectomy (I
approach that is
nephrectomy.[1]
nephrectomy ha
associated with
Efforts to redu
preserving neph
technologies.

With the int
probes, targeted
sible.[2] Tempera
resulting in dir
mation or secon
phase.[3] Histolog
by fibrosis in th
can also be acco
exceeding 60°C
peratures of th
current via a ne
ous CA were rep
their initial seri
colleagues[7] repo
and laparoscop
measure preced

INDICATIO

The indications
cations for nep
have typically b
generally consi
with a small
complex renal
imperative indi
cally or functio
ablative technol
of diseases tha
such as diabet
renal artery ste

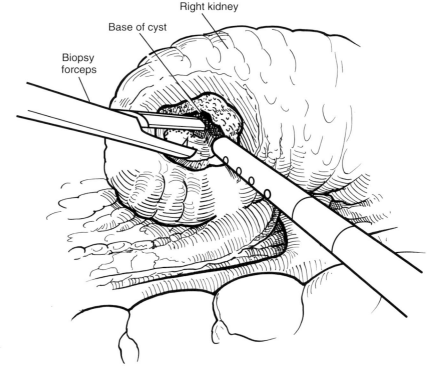

FIGURE 12–13. The base of the cyst is carefully inspected, and biopsy samples are obtained with laparoscopic biopsy forceps.

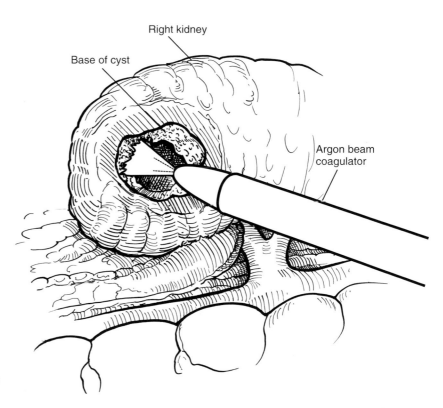

FIGURE 12–14. Argon beam coagulation is used at the cyst base.

cyst with the argon beam coagulator (Fig. 12–14), and place surgical cellulose (e.g., Surgicel, Johnson & Johnson, Inc., Arlington, TX) in the cavity. Take care to avoid inadvertent entry into the collecting system. If injury is suspected, confirm it using retrograde installation of methylene blue through the ureteral catheter. If the collecting system is entered, close it using standard suturing techniques and place a drain either through the lateral port site or via a separate stab incision at the completion of the case (Fig. 12–15). Again, place Surgicel in the cavity, and apply additional fibrin sealant, if needed, to ensure hemostasis and prevent leaks. Bring the colon over the kidney and attach it to the side wall to "re-retroperitonealize" the kidney and drain (Fig. 12–16). If there is no collecting system entry, a drain is not necessary.

REFER

1. Wolf
   Urol 1
2. Bosni
   158:1-
3. Leder
   tion s
4. Wehl
   renal
   136:4
5. Santia
   indete
6. Guazz
   of sim
7. Rober
   of syn
   169, 2

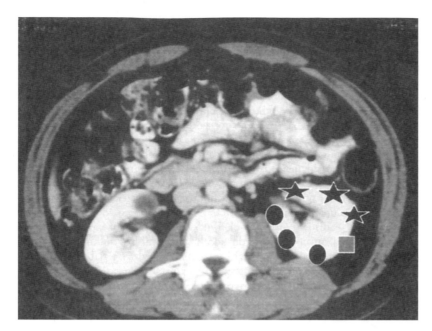

FIGURE 13–3. Anterior tumors (*stars*) are usually best approached by a transperitoneal approach. Tumors (*circles*) are usually best approached with a retroperitoneal approach. The tumor indicated by a *square* is in a location that can be treated with either approach.

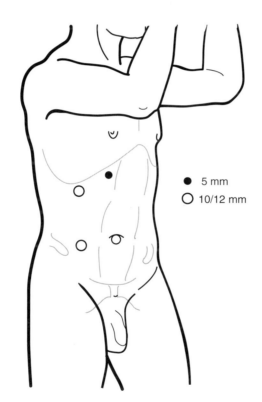

● 5 mm
○ 10/12 mm

FIGURE 13–4. Transperitoneal trocar positions.

num and kocherize. These steps provide visualization of the anterior surface of Gerota's fascia overlying the kidney and anterior hilum. For the retroperitoneal approach, the psoas muscle and the pulsations of the renal artery are usually immediately visible and serve as important anatomic landmarks.

Regardless of approach, enter Gerota's fascia near the tumor. If the patient has significant perirenal fat and the tumor is difficult to discern, laparoscopic US with a flexible probe helps expedite tumor identification. Excise the fat overlying the tumor, and send it for histopathologic examination. Extensively

mobilize the kidney within Gerota's fascia. Renal mobilization allows for passage of a flexible laparoscopic US probe on the surface of the kidney opposite the tumor to optimize imaging and targeting of the tumor. Note the tumor size, margins, vascularity, and proximity to collecting system or hilar structures. Next, percutaneously pass a biopsy device with a 15-gauge Tru-Cut needle (ASAP Biopsy System, Microvasive; Boston Scientific, Watertown, MA) into the tumor and tissue obtain a sample for histopathology.

Laparoscopic Cryoablation

Percutaneously introduce the probes and visually guide them into the tumor. Because the temperature extremes are realized only at the distal aspect of the probes for CA and RFA, skin complications are rare. Targeting tumors is the most challenging component of the procedure and will differentiate success from failure. Initially, collaborating with a radiologist familiar with US images of the kidney may help targeting. With experience, a radiologist is only infrequently required. On rare occasions, tumor identification is very challenging. In these cases, fill the operative field with sterile saline to help improve contact of the flexible laparoscopic probe with the kidney.

Tumor targeting and ablation are critical for success. Depending on tumor size, the number of cryoprobes can vary from one to four. We prefer 1.47-mm IceRods (Galil Medical, Plymouth Meeting, PA), which have been characterized to have an ablative diameter of 1.9 cm.[10] Typically, use a cluster of cryoprobes positioned 1.5 cm apart from one another in a triangular or quadratic configuration to ensure cryolesion overlap. Introduce the IceRods through an external template that is placed on the skin to ensure precise spacing. Mobilize the kidney so that the probes enter the renal parenchyma in a perpendicular manner whenever possible. Grasp the probes with a laparoscopic instrument and insert into the tumor such that they are parallel to each other, thus ensuring proper spacing. Position the flexible laparoscopic US probe to allow imaging of the deepest margin of the tumor. Introduce the IceRods into the tumor under US guidance, and advance them just beyond

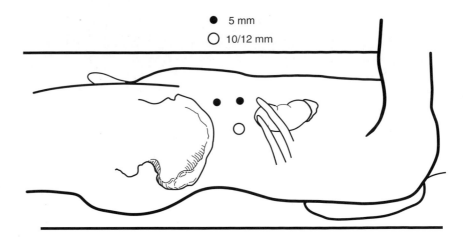

FIGURE 13–5. Retroperitoneal trocar positions.

the deepest margin. Next, perform a double freeze cycle each followed by an active thaw. Continue the first freeze until the iceball extends to a perimeter 1-cm margin beyond the tumor in every direction. Take care to prevent contact of the iceball with critical structures such as the renal vasculature, ureter, renal pelvis, and bowel structures. Mobilize and retract these structures, as needed, to prevent injury. After an appropriate margin has been achieved, perform an active thaw and deploy a second freeze cycle.

After the second freeze cycle, activate an active thaw and remove the IceRods only when they can be twisted gently without resistance. Exercise care not to apply premature force on the IceRods to avert potential fracture of the iceball from the kidney, which may be associated with significant hemorrhage. After removal of the IceRods, hemostasis is typically good and bleeding has not been a problem with these small-caliber probes. Usually, no hemostatic measures are required and we no longer use surgical hemostatics (e.g., fibrin glues or FloSeal). If bleeding does occur, apply gentle pressure for hemostasis.

Laparoscopic Radiofrequency Ablation

Achieve access as described for laparoscopic CA. Percutaneously introduce the probe and enter the tumor perpendicular to the surface of the kidney. Based on tumor size as measured by preoperative CT or MRI and intraoperative US imaging, deploy the tines to a diameter that ensures ablation of the tumor and a 1-cm margin of normal renal tissue. Multiple impedance-based or temperature-based probes are commercially available. Deploy the probes as per protocols, which are delineated in the manufacturer's recommendations. The size of the ablated area is dependent on the diameter of the deployed tines and the activation time. Typically, activation times range from 3 to 8 minutes, and two cycles are performed with a brief interval between cycles to allow cooling. After the tumor ablation is complete, ablate the probe tract while removing the probe from the kidney. This technique minimizes the risk of bleeding and tumor seeding.

Percutaneous Ablation

Administer a general anesthetic or conscious sedation, and position the patient prone in an interventional CT or MRI unit. MRI permits acquisition of sagittal or coronal T1 images to assist in spatial orientation. Position the tip of a 20-gauge

needle just outside the tumor margin to define the eventual probe tract on repeat scans. Perform needle core biopsy of the renal mass along this tract. Advance the CA or RFA probe into the lesion as described for laparoscopic procedures. Obtain repeat scans before ablation to check probe position for adequacy. Perform ablation as described earlier. After ablation, use immediate CT with intravenous contrast to assess for enhancement. Alternatively, MRI demonstrates cryolesions as a signal void on T1-weighted images. Pass absorbable hemostatic material through an introducer after removing the probe to assist hemostasis.[11]

POSTOPERATIVE MANAGEMENT

Patients are quickly advanced to a regular diet as tolerated. A hematocrit is checked in the recovery room and the morning after surgery. Percutaneously administered treatment may permit outpatient care; otherwise, patients are discharged in 23 hours. As per our protocols, patients have follow-up evaluations 1, 3, and 6 months after the procedure with contrast CT or MRI. Then, CT or MRI is obtained every 6 months until 3 years after surgery and then annually. Complete loss of contrast enhancement on follow-up CT or MRI is considered a sign of complete tissue destruction.[4,11] Indeed, we have found that the 3-month imaging follow-up evaluation is the most accurate to determine the success of ablation. Although each urologist must develop a postoperative follow-up plan, initial postoperative imaging at 3 months is suggested at this time.

COMPLICATIONS

Table 13–1 summarizes the complications of CA and RFA reported in the literature. The meta-analysis shows similar complication rates of 10.6% for CA and 13.9% for RFA. In a recent multi-institutional review of CA and RFA procedures, a comparable overall complication rate of 11.1% was reported (14.4% after CA and 7.6% after RFA).[26] The same authors reported similar complication rates between procedures performed laparoscopically (8.9%) and percutaneously (12.2%). The most common complication reported was pain or paresthesias related to the probe site, which was usually self-limited. When compared with LPN, the less technically challenging ablative procedures offer lower complication rates.

TABLE 13–1. COMPLICATIONS OF RENAL CRYOABLATION AND RADIOFREQUENCY ABLATION

Cryoablation				Radiofrequency Ablation			
Reference	Technique	No. of Patients	Morbidity	Reference	Technique	No. of Patients	Morbidity
Rodriguez et al[12]	Three laparoscopic/ four open	7	One pelvic thrombus One CVA	Matsumoto et al[18]	Laparoscopic	28	One UPJ obstruction Two minor
Harmon et al[13]	39 Laparascopic/37 open	76	Six capsular fractures Two prolonged ileus One CVA	DiMarco et al[19]	US/CT guided	66	One UPJ obstruction Two chronic lumbar pain One renal infarct One major hemorrhage
Nadler et al[14]	Laparoscopic	15	One respiratory failure One prolonged ileus	de Baere et al[20]	US/CT guided, 200 W	5	One subcapsular hematoma
Lee et al[15]	Laparoscopic	20	One pancreatic injury	Hwang et al[21]	Nine laparoscopic Eight US/CT guided, 200 W	17	One UPJ obstruction
Shingleton and Sewell[16]	MRI guided	90	One perinephric hematoma Eight minor	Roy-Choudhury et al[22]	US/CT guided, 200 W	8	Two renal infarcts One psoas thermal injury
Colon and Fuchs[17]	Laparoscopic	8	0	Mayo-Smith et al[23]	US/CT guided, 200 W	32	Two perinephric hematomas One probe site skin metastasis
				Su et al[24]	CT guided, 90 W	29	Eight hematomas One thermal hepatic injury One aspiration/death
				Ukimura et al[25]	US/CT guided, 100 W	9	One perinephric hematoma
Overall		216	23 (10.6%)	Overall		194	27 (13.9%)

CT, computed tomography; CVA, cerebrovascular accident; UPJ, ureteropelvic junction; US, ultrasonography.

SUMMARY

Cryoablation and radiofrequency ablation are new and promising technologies for the minimally invasive treatment of small renal cortical neoplasms. With 3- and 5-year follow-up data now demonstrating excellent efficacy, these technologies likely will be increasingly applied to treatment of the small renal mass. Certainly, 10-year follow-up data will help urologists establish the definitive role for these ablative technologies in clinical practice.

Tips and Tricks

■ Tumor location within the kidney and relative to surrounding structures on preoperative imaging indicates whether a laparoscopic or percutaneous approach is prudent.
■ Prone or lateral preoperative imaging for percutaneous procedures determines if intervening structures impede the tract of the ablation probe.
■ High-quality recent (within 3 months) axial imaging (CT or MRI) helps facilitate tumor localization and targeting of ablation probes.
■ Intraoperative real-time laparoscopic US is essential for tumor targeting and, during CA, for monitoring of iceball progression.

■ Extensive mobilization of the kidney during laparoscopic procedures allows the flexible US probe to achieve multiple angles of vision of the tumor and ablation probes.
■ During laparoscopic cases, flooding the operative field with sterile saline may help identify very challenging tumors by improving flexible laparoscopic ultrasound probe contact with the kidney.
■ Both CA and RFA are viable options for the treatment of small renal tumors, less challenging than LPN, and associated with lower complication rates.

REFERENCES

1. Ramani AP, Desai MM, Steinberg AP, et al: Complications of laparoscopic partial nephrectomy in 200 cases. J Urol 173:42–47, 2005.
2. Lutzeyer W, Lumberopoulos S, Breining H: Experimental cryosurgery of the kidney. Langebecks Arch Chir 322:843–847, 1968.
3. Baust J, Gage AA: The molecular basis of cryosurgery. BJU Int 95:1187–1191, 2005.
4. Ogan K, Jacomides L, Dolmatch BL, et al: Percutaneous radiofrequency ablation of renal tumors: Technique, limitations, and morbidity. Urology 60:954–958, 2002.
5. Uchida M, Imaida Y, Sugimoto K, et al: Percutaneous cryotherapy for renal tumors. Br J Urol 75:132–136, 1995.
6. Gill IS, Novick AC, Soble JJ, et al: Laparoscopic renal cryoablation: Initial clinical series. Urology 52:543–551, 1998.

7. Zlotta AR, Wildschutz T, Wood BJ, et al: Radiofrequency interstitial tumor ablation (RITA) is a new modality for treatment of renal cancer: Ex vivo and in vivo experience. J Endourol 11:251–256, 1997.

8. Gettman MT, Bishoff JT, Su LM, et al: Hemostatic laparoscopic partial nephrectomy: Initial experience with the radiofrequency coagulation-assisted technique. Urology 58:8–11, 2001.

9. Pattaras JG, Moore RG, Landman J, et al: Incidence of post-operative adhesion formation after transperitoneal genitourinary laparoscopic surgery. Urology 59: 37–41, 2002.

10. Ames CD, Vanlangendonck R, Venkatesh R, et al: Enhanced renal parenchymal cryoablation with novel 17-gauge cryoprobes. Urology 64:173–175, 2004.

11. Shingleton WB, Sewell PE: Percutaneous renal tumor cryoablation with magnetic resonance imaging guidance. J Urol 165:773–776, 2001.

12. Rodriguez R, Chan DY, Bishoff JT, et al: Renal ablative cryosurgery in selected patients with peripheral renal masses. Urol 55:25–30, 2000.

13. Harmon JD, Parulkar B, Haleblian G, et al: Long-term outcomes of renal cryoablation [abstract]. J Urol 169(suppl):229, 2003.

14. Nadler RB, Kim SC, Rubenstein JN, et al: Laparoscopic renal cryosurgery: The Northwestern experience. J Urol 170:1121–1125, 2003.

15. Lee DI, McGinnis DE, Feld R, et al: Retroperitoneal laparoscopic cryoablation of small renal tumors: Intermediate results. Urol 61:83–88, 2003.

16. Shingleton WB, Sewell PE: Percutaneous renal tumor cryoablation: Results in the first 90 patients [abstract]. J Urol 171(suppl):463, 2004.

17. Colon I, Fuchs GJ: Early experience with laparoscopic cryoablation in patients with small renal tumors and severe comorbidities. J Endourol 17:415–423, 2003.

18. Matsumoto ED, Johnson DB, Ogan K, et al: Laparoscopic radiofrequency ablation of small renal tumors [abstract]. J Urol 171(suppl):127, 2004.

19. DiMarco DS, Farrell MA, Zincke H, et al: Radiofrequency ablation of renal tumors [abstract]. J Urol 171(suppl):129, 2004.

20. de Baere T, Kuoch V, Smayra T, et al: Radiofrequency ablation of renal cell carcinoma preliminary experience. J Urol 167:1961–1964, 2002.

21. Hwang JJ, Walther MM, Pautler SE, et al: Radiofrequency ablation of small renal tumors: Intermediate results. J Urol 171:1814–1818, 2004.

22. Roy-Choudhury SH, Cast JE, Cooksey G, et al: Early experience with percutaneous radiofrequency ablation of small solid renal masses. AJR Am J Roentgenol 180:1055–1061, 2003.

23. Mayo-Smith WW, Dupuy DE, Parikh PM, et al: Imaging-guided percutaneous radiofrequency ablation of solid renal masses: Techniques and outcomes of 38 treatment sessions in 32 consecutive patients. AJR Am J Roentgenol 180:1503–1508, 2003.

24. Su LM, Jarrett TW, Chan DY, et al: Percutaneous computed tomography-guided radiofrequency ablation of renal masses in high surgical risk patients: Preliminary results. Urology 61(suppl):26–33, 2003.

25. Ukimura O, Kawauchi A, Fujito A, et al: Radio-frequency ablation of renal cell carcinoma in patients who were at significant risk. Int J Urol 11:1051–1057, 2004.

26. Johnson DB, Solomon SB, Su LM, et al: Defining the complications of cryoablation and radio frequency ablation of small renal tumors: A multi-institutional review. J Urol 172:874–877, 2004.

CHAPTER 14

Laparoscopic Renal Biopsy

Stephen V. Jackman

Renal biopsy is a crucial tool in the diagnosis of medical disease of the kidney. Histologic information is pivotal in making treatment decisions and providing prognostic information. Ultrasound (US)-guided percutaneous needle biopsy is the current standard for obtaining renal tissue. It has the advantage of being performed under local anesthesia in an outpatient setting. Unfortunately, there is up to a 5% rate of significant hemorrhagic complications.[1]

In instances in which percutaneous biopsy has failed or is considered to pose a high risk, patients are traditionally referred for open renal biopsy. This procedure allows the advantage of obtaining hemostasis and plentiful cortical tissue under direct vision. However, open renal biopsy has the associated morbidity of an incision and general anesthesia. Laparoscopic renal biopsy combines the advantages of open biopsy with the decreased morbidity of a two-port outpatient procedure. General anesthesia is still required.

INDICATIONS AND CONTRAINDICATIONS

The indication for renal biopsy is suspected renal disease, the treatment of which would be influenced by the results of histopathologic tissue analysis. The indications for directly visualized renal biopsy include three categories: failed percutaneous needle biopsy, difficult anatomy, and high risk for bleeding complications.

Anatomic factors that may make a patient unsuitable for percutaneous biopsy include morbid obesity, multiple bilateral cysts, a body habitus that makes positioning impossible, and a solitary functioning kidney. The risk of hemorrhagic complication may outweigh the advantages of percutaneous biopsy in patients who are receiving long-term anticoagulation, have coexistent coagulopathy, or refuse blood transfusion under any circumstance. Laparoscopic renal biopsy is contraindicated in patients with uncorrected coagulopathy, uncontrolled hypertension, or inability to tolerate general anesthesia.

PATIENT PREOPERATIVE EVALUATION AND PREPARATION

Patients undergo routine screening history, physical examination, and blood analyses, including a complete blood count, basic metabolic panel, coagulation panel (prothrombin time, activated partial thromboplastin time), and blood typing with antibody screening. Any problems are evaluated and corrected to the extent possible as determined by the urgency of the biopsy. Additionally, patients must be told to refrain from taking aspirin, nonsteroidal anti-inflammatory drugs (except selective cyclooxygenase-2 inhibitors) and clopidogrel [Plavix]) for 5 to 10 days before their procedure. Patients with bleeding disorders need 2 to 4 units of packed red blood cells crossmatched and available before the start of the procedure.

The patient on long-term anticoagulation therapy is managed in cooperation with the primary physician, nephrologist, or cardiologist. Ideally, if the patient can tolerate cessation of anticoagulation for a short time, the patient stops warfarin 4 to 5 days before admission and undergoes a prothrombin time check the day before surgery. Fresh-frozen plasma can be given if needed just before the procedure. The patient who cannot tolerate cessation of anticoagulation also stops taking warfarin 4 to 5 days before the procedure but must be admitted 2 days before surgery for intravenous anticoagulation. This therapy can be discontinued 6 hours before incision. Alternatively, the patient may be managed as an outpatient with low-molecular-weight heparin injections.

Ideally, the patient can resume the usual oral warfarin dose 24 to 48 hours after surgery, but this must be done cautiously. Closely follow up with patients who require intravenous heparin to ensure that they do not become supratherapeutic.

Patients with thrombocytopenia, which is common in several renal diseases, can receive platelets 30 minutes before incision to boost their platelet count to greater than 50,000 cells/mm^3. Further platelet transfusion is not necessary in the absence of symptomatic bleeding. Uremic patients may benefit from desmopressin acetate (DDAVP) treatment to improve platelet function.

OPERATING ROOM CONFIGURATION AND PATIENT POSITIONING

The surgeon and assistant both stand at the patient's back. Place the video monitor in front of the patient. Position the scrub nurse or technician in front of the patient, caudad to the monitor (Fig. 14–1). In addition to standard laparoscopic equipment, required tools include an optical trocar (Visiport [U.S. Surgical, Norwalk, CT]; Optiview [Ethicon Endo-Surgery, Cincinnati, OH]; or Optical Separator [Applied Medical, Rancho Santa Margarita, CA]), 5-mm two-tooth laparoscopic biopsy forceps, argon beam coagulator, and oxidized regenerated cellulose (Surgicel [Johnson & Johnson, Arlington, TX]).

Place the patient on the operating table in the supine position, then apply antiembolism stockings and sequential com-

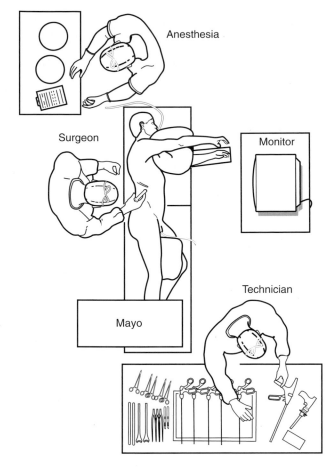

FIGURE 14–1. The surgeon stands behind the patient and a single video monitor is placed in front of the patient. The scrub nurse or technician is located in front of the patient caudad to the monitor.

pression devices. Induce general endotracheal anesthesia, then place an orogastric tube and a urethral catheter. Give from 1 to 2 g of cefazolin for antimicrobial prophylaxis.

Primarily base the choice of which kidney to biopsy for a sample on patient-specific anatomic considerations. A right-sided procedure may be more comfortable for right-handed surgeons, whereas biopsy of the left kidney may involve better working angles due to its higher position. The technique is essentially the same regardless of side.

After inducing anesthesia, carefully roll the patient into the full flank position with the umbilicus over the table break. Fully flex the table to increase the space between the iliac crest and the costal margin. Additionally, raise the kidney rest as needed. Carefully support the head with the headrest, folded sheets, and a head support ring. Align the cervical spine with the thoracic and lumbar spine. Place an axillary roll just below the axilla, and gently extend the arms. Pad the lower elbow with egg crate foam, and place several pillows between the arms.

Securely tape the upper body and arms to the table in position using 3-inch cloth adhesive tape. Use a towel or egg crate foam to protect the skin, upper elbow, and nipples from direct contact with the tape. Some skin contact is often necessary to adequately stabilize the patient.

Flex the lower leg at the hip and knee and pad under the ankle. Leave the upper leg straight and separate it from the lower leg with one or two pillows. Place a standard safety strap around the legs and table at the level of the knees. Securely tape the pelvis in position with more cloth tape, using a towel or egg crate foam over the genitalia for protection. Place grounding pads for electrocautery and the argon beam coagulator on the exposed upper thigh. Then shave, prepare, and drape the patient in standard surgical fashion (Figs. 14–2 and 14–3).

TROCAR PLACEMENT

Retroperitoneal access is identical for either right- or left-sided procedures. Mark the skin midway between the iliac crest and the tip of the 12th rib roughly in the posterior axillary line (Fig. 14–4). Make a 10-mm transverse incision in the skin, and use a small curved hemostat to spread the skin and subcutaneous fat. Place a 0-degree lens with the light on "standby" and focused on the blade of an optical trocar in the incision. Holding the optical trocar perpendicular to the skin and aiming approximately 10 degrees anteriorly, repeatedly fire the blade under direct vision until the retroperitoneum is entered. This requires traversing subcutaneous fat and either the lumbodorsal fascia or the flank musculature (external and internal obliques and the transversus abdominis) (Fig. 14–5). Straying too far anteriorly can result in peritoneal entry or colon injury, whereas posteriorly, the quadratus or psoas muscles can be damaged, resulting in excessive bleeding.

Once the retroperitoneum is entered, remove the Visiport, leaving behind the 12-mm port. Begin CO_2 insufflation at a pressure of 15 to 20 mm Hg. Use blunt dissection with the laparoscope to develop the retroperitoneal space. Anteriorly, sweep the peritoneum medially with the laparoscope, exposing the underside of the transversalis fascia (Fig. 14–6). Once anterior dissection has mobilized the peritoneum medial to the anterior axillary line, place a 5-mm port under direct vision at the same level as the first port (Fig. 14–7). Then use laparoscopic scissors with electrocautery or a Harmonic Scalpel (Ethicon Endo-Surgery, Cincinnati, OH) to assist in completion of retroperitoneal space development. The superior extent of dissection is Gerota's fascia at the level of the lower pole of the kidney.

Open, Hasson-type, entry into the retroperitoneum and balloon dissection is an alternative to the method just described (see Chapter 1, Basic Techniques in Laparoscopic Surgery). The balloon is best placed inside Gerota's fascia before inflation, if possible, for the most efficient access to the kidney.

PROCEDURE

Kidney Exposure and Biopsy

Once both the camera and working trocar are in position and an adequate working space has been created, direct the instruments away from the midline toward the lower pole of the kidney (Fig. 14–8). Locate the kidney by palpation and sharp dissection through Gerota's fascia. The change to a darker-yellow fat upon entry into Gerota's fascia helps identify the kidney (Fig. 14–9). In morbidly obese or other difficult situa-

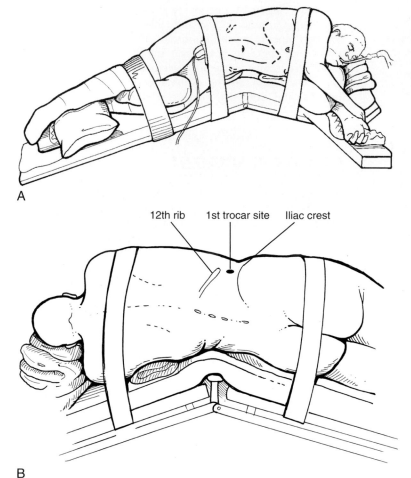

A

12th rib   1st trocar site   Iliac crest

B

FIGURE 14–2. *A,* The patient is placed into a full flank position with the umbilicus over the table break. The table is fully flexed to increase the space between the iliac crest and the costal margin. Additionally, the kidney rest may be raised as needed. The head is carefully supported with the headrest, folded sheets, and a head support ring. The lower elbow should be padded with egg crate foam, and several pillows are placed between the arms. The chest, pelvis, thigh, lower leg, and arms are securely taped with 3-inch cloth adhesive tape. *B,* The cervical spine should be aligned with the thoracic and lumbar spine. An axillary roll is placed just below the axilla, and the arms are gently extended.

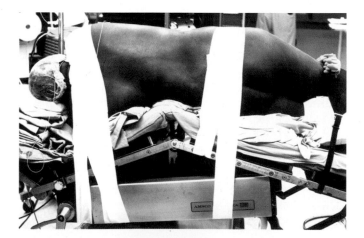

FIGURE 14–3. Patient positioned for laparoscopic renal biopsy.

tions, preoperative transcutaneous or intraoperative US may be valuable in localizing the kidney.

Once Gerota's fascia is incised, sweep the perirenal fat aside to expose an approximately 2 × 2 cm area of the lower pole (Fig. 14–10). Use the 5-mm two-tooth biopsy forceps to take two or three good cortical renal biopsy specimens (Fig. 14–11). Place these in saline and transport them immediately to pathology for confirmation that adequate kidney tissue was obtained. Do not place the specimens in formalin; important information will be lost if the specimens are placed in formalin before processing. Frozen section or gross inspection under a dissecting microscope will confirm the presence of renal tissue. The pathologist can then place the tissue in the appropriate fixative for analysis.

Hemostasis and Closure

Obtain hemostasis with the argon beam coagulator. During activation of the argon beam, it is important to vent the increased pressure created in the retroperitoneum by the flow of argon gas (Fig. 14–12). While awaiting pathologic confirmation of sufficient specimen, lower the insufflation pressure to 5 mm Hg for at least 5 minutes and inspect the entire retroperitoneum for hemostasis. Treat persistent bleeding from the biopsy site with repeated argon beam coagulation. Pack oxidized cellulose (Surgicel) into the biopsy site and apply direct pressure (Fig. 14–13). Other adjuncts to hemostasis are needed rarely; these include various fibrin glues, matrix hemostatic sealant (FloSeal, Baxter, Fremont, CA), and surgical adhesives (BioGlue, CryoLife, Kennesaw, GA). Clip oozing vessels that are distant from the biopsy site with a 5-mm clip applier instead

Text continued on page 169

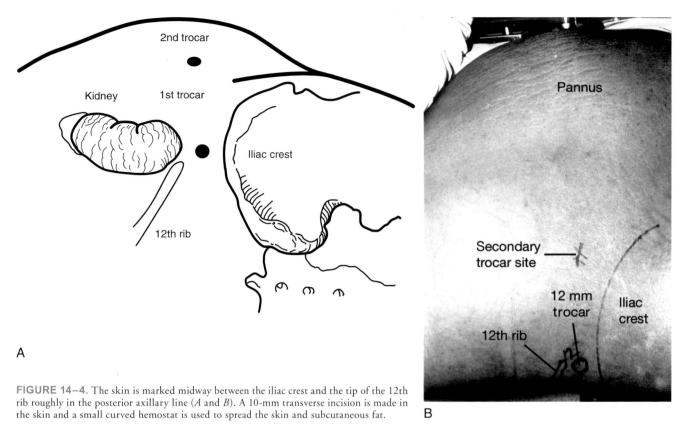

A

B

FIGURE 14–4. The skin is marked midway between the iliac crest and the tip of the 12th rib roughly in the posterior axillary line (*A* and *B*). A 10-mm transverse incision is made in the skin and a small curved hemostat is used to spread the skin and subcutaneous fat.

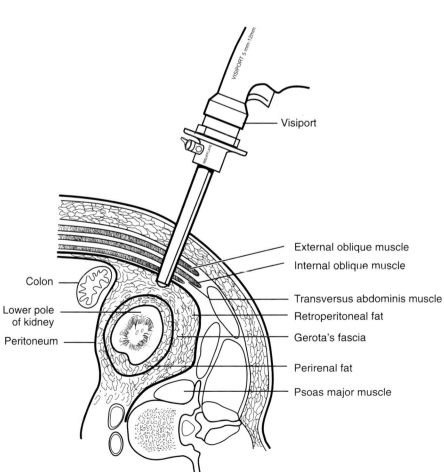

FIGURE 14–5. Use of an optical trocar such as the Visiport (U.S. Surgical, Norwalk, CT) allows the trocar to be advanced through the fascial layers into the retroperitoneum under direct vision.

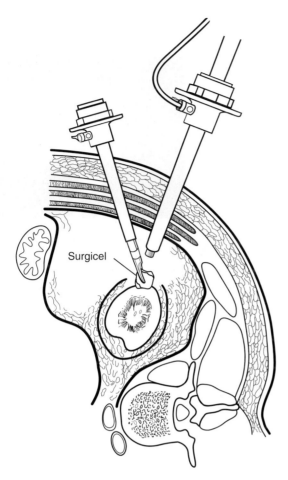

FIGURE 14–13. Surgicel is passed down the 5-mm port and placed over the area of the biopsy.

REFERENCES

1. Wickre CG, Golper TA: Complications of percutaneous needle biopsy of the kidney. Am J Nephrol 2:173, 1982.
2. Shetye KR, Kavoussi, Ramakumar S, et al: Laparoscopic renal biopsy: A 9-year experience. BJU Int 91:817-820, 2003.

CHAPTER 15

Laparoscopic Pyeloplasty

Itay Y. Vardi
Sam B. Bhayani

Laparoscopic pyeloplasty has evolved into a new standard of care for the treatment of ureteropelvic junction obstruction. Since it was introduced in the early 1990s,[1,2] the laparoscopic approach has maintained the high efficacy of open surgery without the coincident morbidity of the open incision. Additionally, the approach is favored over endopyelotomy[3,4] because complex reconstruction can be performed, even in the presence of aberrant crossing vessels.[5] The surgery does require intracorporeal suturing skills, which may be perfected in an inanimate trainer before operative intervention.[6]

INDICATIONS AND CONTRAINDICATIONS

The indications for laparoscopic pyeloplasty include any patient who has documented ureteropelvic junction obstruction.[7] Preoperative three-dimensional computed tomography (CT) reconstruction of the ureteropelvic junction (UPJ) may allow visualization of crossing vessels,[8] but is not necessary in all cases. There are few contraindications to laparoscopic pyeloplasty. Besides routine surgical contraindications (medical comorbidities, multiple surgeries or infections, renal or ureteral adhesions, uncorrected coagulopathies), the operation may be performed in virtually any age patient and with any anatomic abnormality.[9] Crossing vessels, renal stones, and duplicated collecting systems can all be addressed laparoscopically. Laparoscopic pyeloplasty may also be performed after failed endopyelotomy, failed open pyeloplasty, or even failed laparoscopic pyeloplasty.[10,11]

PATIENT PREOPERATIVE EVALUATION AND PREPARATION

In assessing the degree of obstruction, a diuretic renal scan may help quantify blockage and residual function. An intravenous urogram or retrograde pyelogram may help define anatomic considerations before reconstruction. A CT angiogram or three-dimensional reconstruction of the UPJ may reveal anterior crossing arteries or veins that will require dismembered pyeloplasty and transposition of the vessels.[8,12] None of these studies, however, is absolutely compulsory because none of them is likely to change the need for surgical intervention. Nevertheless, the studies may produce a surgical map of the field, thus allowing for less intraoperative speculation.[12]

Obtain informed consent from the patient, and discuss major risks, benefits, and alternatives. Discuss general surgical risks and other risks more germane to the procedure, including the possibility of urine leak, injury to surrounding structures, failure of surgery, migration of stents and drains, open conversion, bleeding, loss of kidney function, and nephrectomy.

Patients may have existing indwelling stents from the diagnosis of obstruction and pain. Typically, indwelling stents may cause ureteral edema and thickening, and identification of the UPJ may be difficult. Consider removing the stent 1 week before surgery if the patient can tolerate this intervention.

Give the patient a bottle of magnesium citrate and clear liquids the day before surgery. This bowel preparation, although not completely necessary, allows decompression of the intestines and may help in visualization during dissection. A negative urine culture is needed or antibiotics are given at the time of surgery. After induction of general anesthesia, place an orogastric tube. Perform flexible or rigid cystoscopy and place a stent into the affected kidney. Use a long stent (7 Fr × 28 cm) so that it does not migrate out of the bladder during reconstruction. Perform a retrograde pyelogram if it is indicated. Place a urethral catheter, and reposition the patient for the pyeloplasty.

OPERATING ROOM CONFIGURATION AND PATIENT POSITIONING

The operating room is configured so that the surgeon and staff have excellent views of the laparoscopic surgical monitors (Fig. 15–1).

Positioning can be performed in a variety of methods. If a difficult dissection is anticipated, position the patient over the break in the table in case open conversion is needed. Place the patient into the full flank position (90 degrees) or the modified flank position (60 degrees, supported by a gel roll). Place the arms high so that they do not interfere with suturing (Fig. 15–2). No flexion is necessary in most cases. Consider adding an axillary roll and ensure adequate padding is used.

TROCAR PLACEMENT

Insert a Veress needle and establish a pneumoperitoneum. Place a 10/12-mm trocar at the umbilicus, a 5-mm trocar 6 to 8 cm superior to the umbilicus, and a 10/12-mm trocar 6 to 8 cm below the umbilical trocar. Place all trocars in the midline; this positioning facilitates ergonomic suturing (Fig. 15–3).

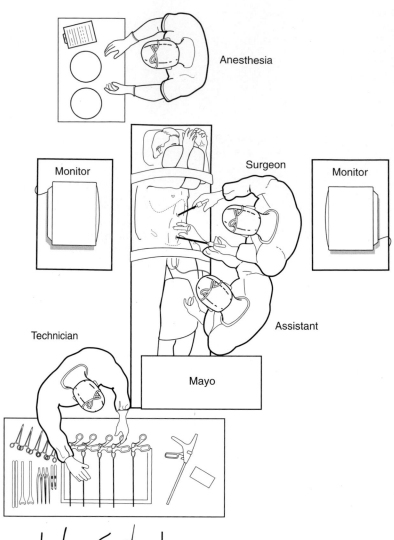

FIGURE 15–1. To allow visualization of the procedure by all members of the surgical team, the surgeon and assistant stand on the side contralateral to the pathology. The scrub nurse or technician stands on the opposite side to help with management of instrumentation.

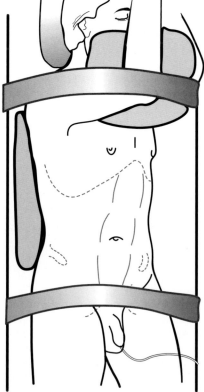

FIGURE 15–2. The umbilicus should be centered at the table break in the event that an open repair would be performed. An axillary role is placed under the lower arm, which is brought out perpendicular to the patient. The arms are then positioned in a "praying position" near the patient's head and separated by a small pillow. The contralateral lower knee is bent at a 90-degree position and the ipsilateral leg is kept straight with pillows or foam placed in between them. Wide cloth tape is placed across the upper shoulder/arm and hip and secured to the operative table.

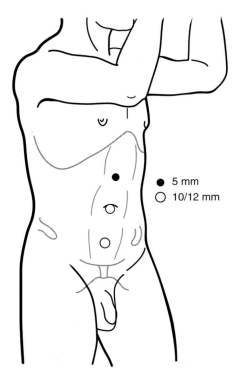

FIGURE 15–3. Trocar placement includes three midline trocars. A 10-mm trocar is placed at the umbilicus. The second port (5 mm) is placed midway between the xiphoid process and the umbilicus. A third trocar is located midway between the umbilicus and the symphysis pubis.

PROCEDURE

Use a 30-degree lens throughout the operation. Reflect the colon using standard laparoscopic techniques, similar to a radical nephrectomy, and identify the ureter. Take care not to mobilize the ureter aggressively because it is necessary to preserve the periureteric blood supply.

Expose the ureter only at the UPJ. The area can be easily found because the pelvis is typically hydronephrotic and the stented ureter can be felt with laparoscopic graspers. The gonadal vein may be mistaken for the ureter, and palpation of the structure may clarify the structure's identity. Take care in dissection of the UPJ because a crossing vessel may be present (Fig. 15–4). Once the UPJ is identified and crossing vessels are recognized, free the renal pelvis from its peripelvic attachments near the UPJ. This allows mobilization of the pelvis and proximal ureter for the anastamosis. Importantly, during the dissection of the UPJ, avoid clips because they could erode into the repair. Control bleeding with energy sources (ultrasonic shears, bipolar cautery, monopolar cautery, and so on), but avoid direct use of energy on the ureter. Control oozing at the cut edge with the sutures during repair.

Hynes-Anderson Dismembered Pyeloplasty

Once a crossing vessel is suspected during preoperative imaging or observed during the procedure itself, a Hynes-Anderson dismembered pyeloplasty is the treatment of choice.[5,13] This approach can also be used in virtually any UPJ obstruction.

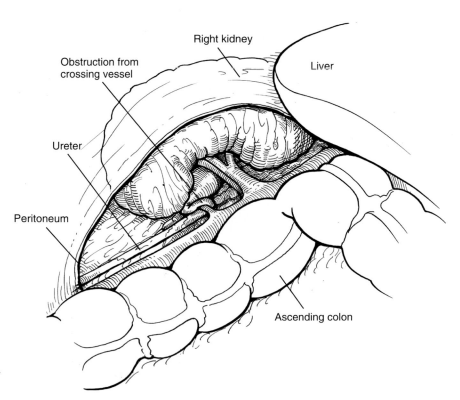

FIGURE 15–4. After the colon is reflected, the ureter is identified at the lower pole of the kidney. A crossing vessel is identified causing obstruction at the level of the ureteropelvic junction.

A segmental renal vessel can be identified in close proximity to the UPJ in up to 60% of patients, and its anterior position may be the cause of the obstruction. Perform the anastamosis between the ureter and the renal pelvis anterior to the vascular obstructing component.

When the renal pelvis is identified, mobilize it along with a small portion of the proximal ureter. Take care not to damage the small vessels supplying the pelvis because, theoretically, it may provide better viability of the anastomosis.

Make a circumferential incision over the renal pelvis above the anastomotic area (Fig. 15–5) and insert the stent. Complete the incision around the stent and along the renal pelvis wall. Take down redundant tissue to enable better approximation and technical results. Distally transect the UPJ using laparoscopic scissors and either remove the ring of ureteral obstructing tissue or incorporate it in the spatulation. Take care not to damage the ureteral stent during this manipulation. Make a 1-cm spatulation incision along the lateral or posterior wall of the proximal ureter. Spatulate the renal pelvis, if needed. Place a 4-0 polyglactin stitch at the tip of the spatulated ureter and then through the renal pelvis.

Once this knot is tied or secured with a Vicryl clip, use this stay suture to assist in applying interrupted sutures along the posterior pyelotomy, tying each knot outside of the urinary tract. These 4-0 sutures can also be placed with the EndoStitch laparoscopic suturing device (Auto Suture, Norwalk, CT)[14] (Figs. 15–6 and 15–7). Once the posterior wall is completed, insert the stent inside the renal pelvis and tailor the anterior portion of the renal pelvis to the spatulated ureter with interrupted 4-0 sutures.

Another method for the pyelotomy closure that is used today is a continuous closure using a double-armed, knotted suture.[15] Tie the sutures at their free end with a simple knot and drive each needle outside-in on the renal pelvis. One suture runs along the posterior wall continuously and the other runs over the anterior wall. Tie them together at the end, outside of the system, with a knot or a Lapra-Ty Vicryl clip (Ethicon Endosurgery Inc, Cincinnati, OH)[14] (Fig. 15–8).

Foley Y-V Pyeloplasty

Use this approach in a small renal pelvis with a high inserted ureter and no crossing vessels. Make a wide-based V-shaped incision over the anterior aspect of the renal pelvis using the laparoscopic scissors (Fig. 15–9). Continue along with a vertical incision through the anterior proximal ureter, as low as 1 cm below the obstructed area. Using a 4-0 polyglactin suture, approximate the tip of the V shape to the apex of the proximal ureter incision. First, suture the medial arm of the V shape with interrupted 4-0 sutures using EndoStitch or standard knots, then insert the ureteral stent into the renal pelvis and close the anterior arm of the V shape with interrupted suturing.

Fenger Non-Dismembered Pyeloplasty

Use this approach with a small-sized renal pelvis and no crossing vessels. The procedure uses the Heineke-Mikulicz principle of a longitudinal incision closed in a transverse fashion. Compared to the procedures previously described, less suturing is needed, thus a shorter operative time is required. Make one long incision with laparoscopic scissors along the anterior renal pelvis and proximal ureter (Fig. 15–10), ending about 1 cm below the obstructed area. Place a 4-0 polyglactin suture from the superior apex of the incision on the renal pelvis, and approach to the inferior apex of the incision on the proximal ureter. Then use three to four interrupted sutures on each side for the transverse closure of the incision.

Take care not to damage the internal ureteral stent with the closure of the incision. With this approach there is no need to free the stent outside of the renal pelvis.

There is some debate as to whether or not this approach is as efficacious as a dismembered pyeloplasty.

Drain Placement

Leave a closed bulb suction drain in close proximity to the anastomotic area, preferably in a posterior position. A 7-Fr or 10-Fr Jackson-Pratt drain is commonly used.

Introduce the drain intra-abdominally through one of the laparoscopic ports (Fig. 15–11). Then make a new stab incision at the lateral abdominal wall and extract the drain outside the abdomen using a small hemostat. Alternatively, pass a drain with a sharpened spike into the retroperitoneum under direct vision, toward a trocar advanced deep into the abdomen, and toward the sharpened spike; pull the drain into the trocar with a spoon forceps. A retroperitoneal position for the drain is preferred because urinomas can drain posteriorly when the patient is recovering in the supine position. Use a nonabsorbable skin stitch to secure the drain.

POSTOPERATIVE MANAGEMENT

A 48-hour admission is typical. However, because urine leaks into the peritoneal cavity during the reconstruction, bowel may be irritated. As a result, the patient may have a slower return of normal bowel function and more postoperative pain compared with laparoscopic nephrectomy patients. Remove the orogastric tube at the end of the procedure. Give clear liquids the night of surgery and advance diet as tolerated.

Some give oral antibiotics throughout the stented period, but most give oral antibiotics only 2 to 3 days before stent removal. Take out the urethral catheter after 48 hours. It is mandatory to closely measure the drain output once the urinary catheter is removed. If this output does not increase in the 8 to 12 hours after catheter removal, remove the drain and discharge the patient.

Suspect anastomotic leak if an increased amount of urine (creatinine level at the drain fluid is higher than the plasma creatinine) is measured in the retroperitoneal drain after urinary catheter removal. Reinsert the catheter into the bladder until the drain output is no longer uriniferous. This may take up to 1 to 2 weeks. Consider the possibility of an obstructed or malpositioned stent if drain output is high with the catheter in place. A CT scan can help in assessment of stent positioning.

Leave the stent in place for 3 to 4 weeks. Consider a diuretic renal scan 6 weeks after surgery and every 4 to 6 months for 2 years. Failures usually occur within the first year postoperatively.[10,11]

Text continued on page 183

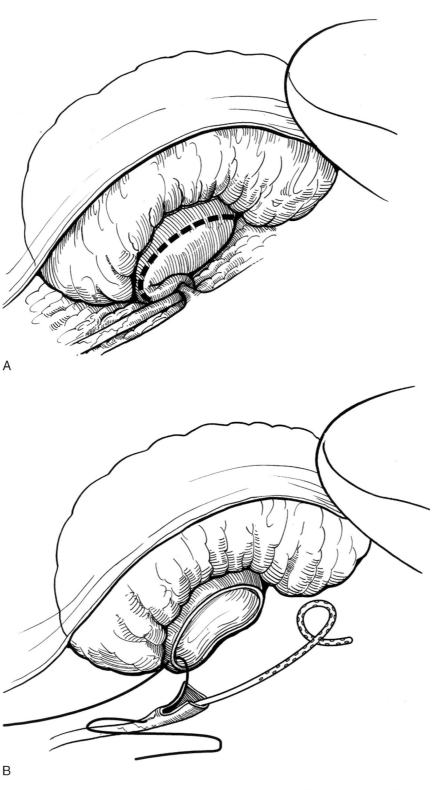

A

B

FIGURE 15–5. *A*, An incision is made on the dilated pelvis to transect the ureteropelvic junction. Care is taken to avoid cutting the stent. *B*, The ureter and pelvis are placed anterior to the crossing vessel. The redundant pelvis and stenotic ureteropelvic junction have been excised and the proximal ureter spatulated. The first suture has been placed from the apex of the spatulated ureter to the most dependent portion of the renal pelvis.

Continued

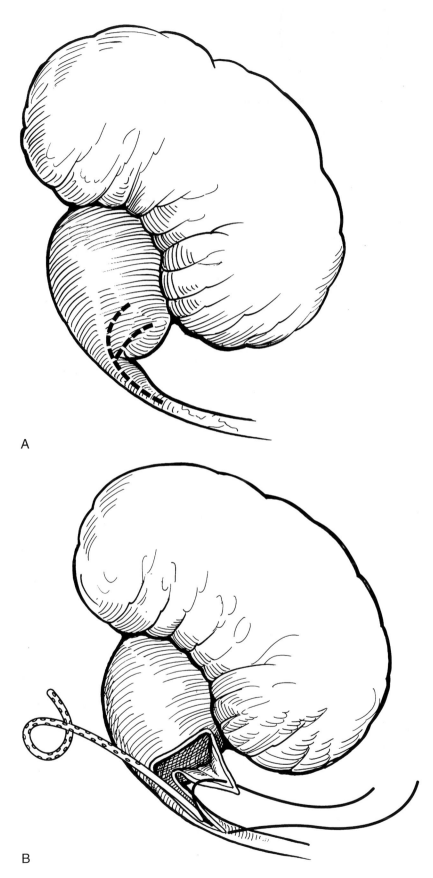

A

B

FIGURE 15–9. *A,* An incision is made in the pelvis extending down on to the ureter through its insertion into the pelvis. A V is formed with arms equal in length to the incision over the ureter. *B,* A 4-0 absorbable suture is passed with the EndoStitch though the apex of the V and the apex of the ureteral incision.

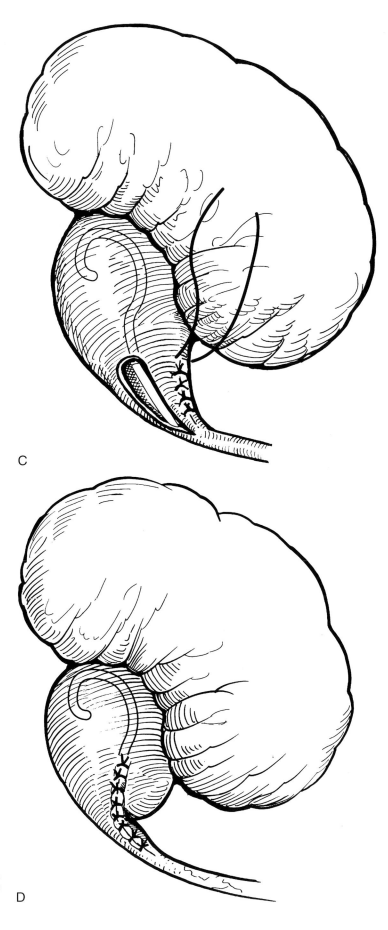

FIGURE 15–9, cont'd. *C,* The inside of the V incision is closed with a running suture. *D,* The anterior incision is closed with 4-0 absorbable suture in an interrupted or running fashion to complete the repair.

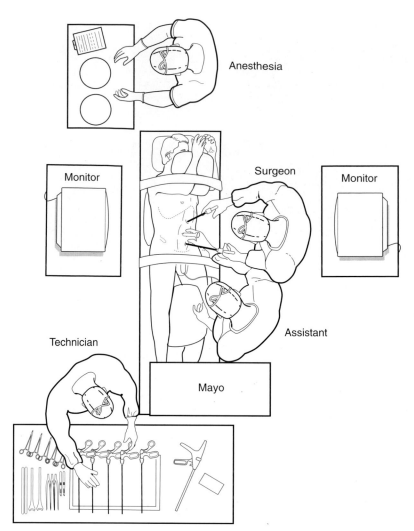

FIGURE 16–2. The operating room is configured so that all personnel can view the procedure.

renal pelvis after diuretic is more an estimation of the extent of impaired ureteral peristalsis than a function of extrinsic obstruction. This can be observed equally during ureteral stent placement. For the most part, the guidewire and stent can be advanced without resistance.

Our preoperative preparation begins 10 days before surgery, when patients stop taking all aspirin-containing products. An updated history, physical examination, laboratory work (including urinalysis and urine culture), chest radiograph, and electrocardiogram are performed within 7 days of the procedure. The day before surgery, patients take 16 ounces of oral magnesium citrate at 3:00 PM with clear liquids to follow until midnight. Patients arrive in the preoperative holding area with an empty stomach except for blood pressure medication and half their usual morning dose of insulin. All patients already had either percutaneous nephrostomy tubes or internal ureteral stents placed at the time of diagnosis.

OPERATING ROOM CONFIGURATION AND PATIENT POSITIONING

The operating team stands on the contralateral side of the affected ureter, looking over the patient directly at the video tower or boom. Place the electrocautery equipment,

compression-stocking pump, and body warmer at the foot of the bed. Bring the suction-irrigator off the head of the bed. The surgical assistant stands caudad to, and the scrub nurse stands opposite, the operating surgeon (Fig. 16–2).

We perform our procedure through a transabdominal approach. Place patient in a supine position. After induction of general endotracheal anesthesia, place 6-French double-J ureteral stents using a flexible cystoscope, and confirm the position with fluoroscopy.

Place a Foley catheter, antiembolism stockings, sequential compression devices, and lower body–warming blanket. Tuck the arms and firmly secure the patient to the table. Securing the patient is very important because of the need to tilt the bed to an extreme angle to facilitate bowel mobilization (Fig. 16–3).

TROCAR PLACEMENT

Trocar placement is dependent on the distal and proximal extent of the fibrotic process and ureteral involvement. We use four 12-mm trocars. Place them in the midline beginning at the subxyphoid position and separated by 8 to 10 cm, depending on the patient's size (Fig. 16–4).

Step-by-Step Procedure

Using a Veress needle through the umbilicus, insufflate the abdominal cavity with CO_2 to 15 cm pressure. Make a 10-mm incision approximately 2 cm superior to the umbilicus. Use a Kelly clamp to spread the subcutaneous tissue off the rectus sheath. Use a Visiport (U.S. Surgical, Norwalk, CT) with the 12-mm trocar and a 0-degree lens to enter the abdominal cavity. With the Visiport, it is important to use blunt downward pressure to reach each fascial plane. Then deploy the blade parallel to the visualized fascial fibers. Do not use excessive downward pressure because it can lead to inadvertent laceration of the bowel wall or mesenteric fat. Discard the Visiport device, and fully inspect the abdominal cavity for evidence of adhesions. Place the three additional trocars under direct vision. Secure each trocar in place at the appropriate depth with a 2-0 silk stay suture.

Tilt the operative table 45 degrees toward the operating team to facilitate mobilization of the bowel. We begin with the three superior ports and the 30-degree lens. Using blunt Maryland dissectors and the suction-irrigator, move the bowel away from the lateral side wall to expose the white line of Toldt in its entirety. At this point, it is essential to have a mental map of the extent of the dissection that will be necessary to completely release the ureter. Incise the white line with EndoShears using a combination of sharp dissection and electrocautery beginning at the iliac vessels and extending superiorly to the inferior margin of the kidney. Keeping a generous lateral sleeve of peritoneum on the bowel will facilitate the intraperitonealization of the ureter. At the inferior margin of the kidney, swing the dissection medially but just lateral to the presumed location of the renal hilum. Then carry this incision superiorly past the apex of the kidney and just lateral to the splenic hilum. On the right, follow the course of the colon around the hepatic flexure and then diagonally to the renal hilum. The dissection needs to extend only 2 cm above the renal hilum on the right.

Moving back to the caudal extent of the incision, identify the margin between mesenteric fat and retroperitoneal fat. Blunt dissection is usually adequate to mobilize the bowel medially. Once the fibrotic process is encountered, the plane of dissection becomes indistinct. Continue superiorly with the easily accomplished mobilization until with spleen has been released. This will allow the spleen to fall to a medial position, bringing along the splenic flexure of the colon.

Frame-shift the instruments to the lowest three trocars and continue the dissection below the level of the iliac vessels. Once the ureter is encountered at a position outside the fibrotic process, free the ureter of attachment and dissect it to the point of entry into the fibrosis. The renal pelvis is rarely involved and consequently is an excellent place to start the dissection (Fig. 16–5). Place a vessel loop or umbilical tape around the ureter and secure the ends together with a clip. This can then be used to manipulate the ureter in a relatively atraumatic fashion (Fig. 16–6).

At this point, the retroperitoneal mass must be exposed adequately. Obtain a series of incisional biopsies, and send them for pathologic frozen sectioning. Take care to avoid the hidden great vessels and involved ureter. A pathologic report of no malignancy allows the case to proceed as planned. Then follow the ureter in a slow and meticulous fashion into the fibrotic mass. Advance a right angle along and superficial to

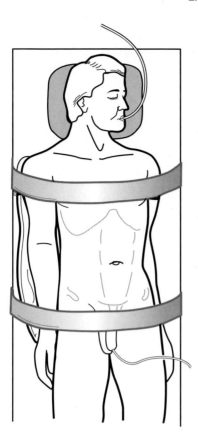

FIGURE 16–3. The patient is positioned in the supine position and secured with wide tape at the hips and shoulders to prevent slipping during rotation of the table.

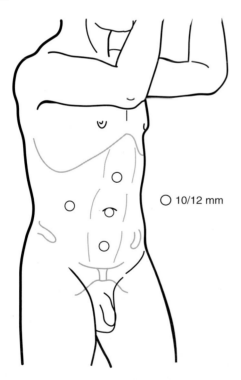

○ 10/12 mm

FIGURE 16–4. Trocar placement for laparoscopic ureterolysis. Two 10-mm midline ports are used. A 10-mm trocar is placed at the umbilicus. The second port is located midway between the xiphoid process and the umbilicus. A third trocar is placed between the pubis symphysis and the umbilicus. A fourth trocar is located lateral to the rectus in line with the umbilicus for retraction or aspiration.

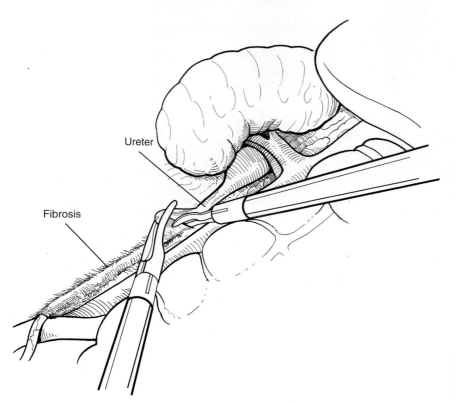

Ureter

Fibrosis

FIGURE 16–5. Once the colon is reflected, the proximal ureter is identified. Using sharp dissection, the ureter is freed circumferentially above the area of fibrosis.

the trajectory of the ureter; this will facilitate division of the mass.

It is tempting to stay right on the ureter, but do not; although this is an easier plane to follow, the result will be a devascularized ureter. This path also increases the risk of creating ureterotomies or, worse, a complete transection of the ureter. It is vitally important to avoid all forms of electrocautery during this part of the dissection. The depth of heat penetration will vary, thus putting the ureter at great risk.

Once the superior margin of the ureteral entrapment has been reached, continue mobilization of the ureter an additional 2 to 3 cm. Fully inspect the ureter along its length. In the best of hands, this is a difficult dissection that often results in multiple ureterotomies. It is vitally important to identify and repair each hole with a 4-0 Monocryl suture.

Intraperitonealization requires careful planning to both avoid ureteral kinking and to ensure isolation from the fibrotic mass. Close the trough that is left in the fibrotic mass after the ureter has been freed with suture or clips (Fig. 16–7). Bring the lateral sleeve of peritoneum that is attached to the bowel under the ureter and affix it to the psoas fascia. The wider this sleeve of tissue, the less ureteral kinking will occur from the bowel now encroaching directly on the renal pelvis. Suture the sleeve along its entire length. We use a 4-0 EndoStitch in a running fashion to achieve this goal. If desired, mobilize a piece of omentum, place it under the ureter, and secure it with a suture (Fig. 16–8).

With the repair complete, inspect and desufflate the abdomen, remove the trocars, and close the fascia with 0-0 Vicryl suture.

POSTOPERATIVE MANAGEMENT

Postoperatively, patients are allowed clear liquids that are advanced to a regular diet as tolerated. For pain management, they are given morphine-based patient-controlled analgesia. The Foley catheter is typically removed once the patient is ambulating and able to comfortably get to the bathroom. Pain management is transitioned to oral narcotics the afternoon of postoperative day 1. Most patients are ready for discharge to home the afternoon of postoperative day 2.

The ureteral stent remains in place for 4 weeks postoperatively. This can be removed in the clinic. Patients are followed with laboratory tests and imaging 2 weeks after the removal of the stent and then on a 6-month basis for 2 years.

COMPLICATIONS

The general complications that can occur with all laparoscopic procedures are discussed elsewhere.

The difficulty of the procedure cannot be understated. The density of the fibrotic process dictates how challenging the dissection will be. Although management of ureteral injury is straightforward and follows usual principles, remember that by virtue of the disease, these are frail patients with multiple comorbidities. They often have an element of renal insufficiency. Consequently, these patients may not be able to tolerate a bowel interposition graft if the ureter is substantially injured or, worse, devascularized.

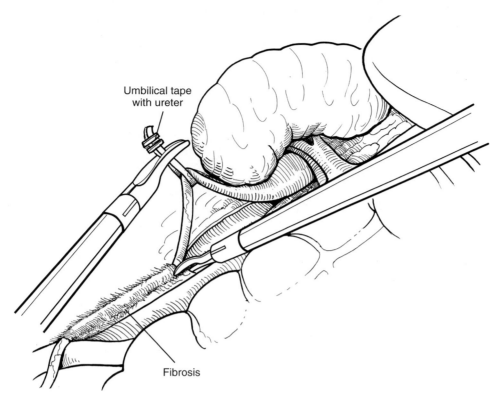

FIGURE 16–6. Traction via a clipped 6-cm piece of umbilical tape aids in dissection. As the ureter is elevated, scissors are used to open the dense fibrosis surrounding the ureter.

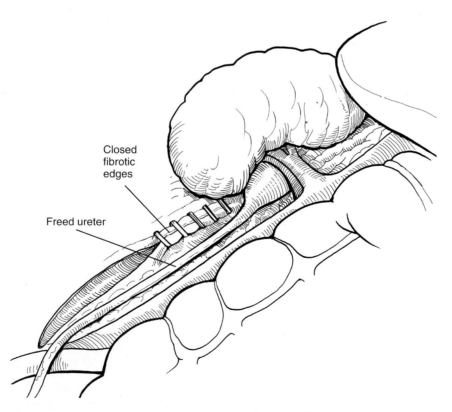

FIGURE 16–7. Reapproximating the peritoneum posteriorly with clips or a suture intraperitonealizes the ureter.

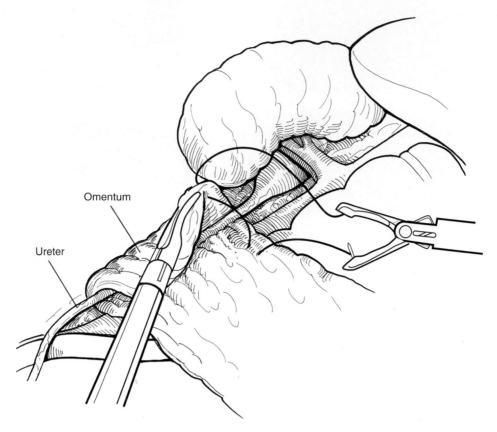

Omentum

Ureter

FIGURE 16–8. A flap of omentum from the transverse colon can be placed under the ureter to protect the ureter from being entrapped in fibrosis and causing obstruction.

Long-term complications include ureteral stricture, ureteral kinking, and reinvolvement of the ureter in the fibrotic mass. Stricture and kinking are primarily a result of surgical technique. With regard to reinvolvement of the ureter in the mass, some have advocated a combined therapeutic approach with the judicious use of long-term low-dose steroids.

SPECIAL INSTRUMENTS

We use a standard laparoscopic tray for this procedure. In that tray are 5-mm instruments: two Maryland dissectors, a short- and long-tip right angle, EndoShears, a suction-irrigator, and an EndoStitch device. Occasionally, we use a lap paddle to assist in bowel retraction.

Tips and Tricks

- Place four 12-mm trocars in the midline to facilitate the cephalad and caudal dissections.
- Leave a wide sleeve on the lateral aspect of the large bowel when incising the white line of Toldt.
- Pay close attention to the lie of the ureter when beginning the superior intraperitonealization. This will reduce the risk of kinking the proximal ureter.

RETROCAVAL URETER

Retrocaval ureter is a rare congenital anomaly that occurs in 1 in 1000 live births. The condition occurs when the infrarenal vena cava develops from the right posterior cardinal vein rather than from the right supracardinal vein. The end result is a proximal ureter that wraps from posterior cephalad to anterior caudad around the vena cava. The condition is limited to the right side, except in rare cases of vena caval duplication. When the retrocaval position leads to proximal hydronephrosis through compression, patients may become symptomatic.

In 1994, Baba and associates[9] described the first laparoscopic repair of a circumcaval ureter. Performed in a 54-year-old man, the procedure followed closely the principles of a dismembered pyeloplasty. They trimmed redundant ureter and performed a primary end-to-end spatulated anastomosis. Numerous descriptions of the retroperitoneal approach exist in the literature.[10–17]

INDICATIONS AND CONTRAINDICATIONS

The relative indications and contraindications to surgically managing these cases with a laparoscopic approach mimic those outlined for the management of ureteropelvic junction obstruction.

PATIENT PREOPERATIVE EVALUATION AND PREPARATION

Evaluation of a patient with suspected retrocaval ureter begins with a complete history and physical examination. Important elements of the history include timing, onset, duration, and description of symptoms. Patients often describe intermittent colicky flank pain, and often the symptoms are worse immediately after ingesting liquids or medications with diuretic properties. The physical examination may demonstrate a large mass in the right upper quadrant, but as with ureteropelvic junction, this finding is relatively uncommon.

The laboratory evaluation focuses on quantification of overall renal function. However, a complete blood cell count, serum electrolytes, urinalysis, and urine culture are important.

The radiologic study of choice has traditionally been the intravenous pyelogram. This will demonstrate a classic reverse J- or S-shape deformity. In addition to anatomic information, the intravenous pyelogram provides a crude estimation of the degree of obstruction (Fig. 16–9).

Our studies of choice are a spiral CT of the abdomen and pelvis with contrast and a MAG3 diuretic renal scan. These two studies provide us with accurate information regarding the position and course of the ureter relative to the inferior vena cava. The nuclear medicine scan provides an objective measure of obstruction and renal split function. Patients with less than 15% function on the affected side may be better managed with a laparoscopic nephrectomy.

Our preoperative preparation of these patients mimics that described for RPF patients.

OPERATING ROOM CONFIGURATION AND PATIENT POSITIONING

The operating team stands on the side contralateral to the affected ureter looking over the patient directly at the video tower/boom. Place the electrocautery equipment, compression-stocking pump, and body warmer at the foot of the bed. Bring the suction irrigator off the head of the bed. The surgical assistant stands cephalad of, and the scrub nurse stands with the table caudad to, the operating surgeon (see Fig. 16–2).

We perform our procedure through a transabdominal approach. Place the patient in a supine position. Induce general endotracheal anesthesia. Using a flexible cystoscope, place a 6-French double-J ureteral stent and confirm the position with fluoroscopy.

Place a Foley catheter, antiembolism stockings, sequential compression devices, and lower body–warming blanket. Tuck the arms, and firmly secure the patient to the operative table (Fig. 16–10). Securing the patient is very important because of the need to tilt the bed to an extreme angle to facilitate bowel mobilization.

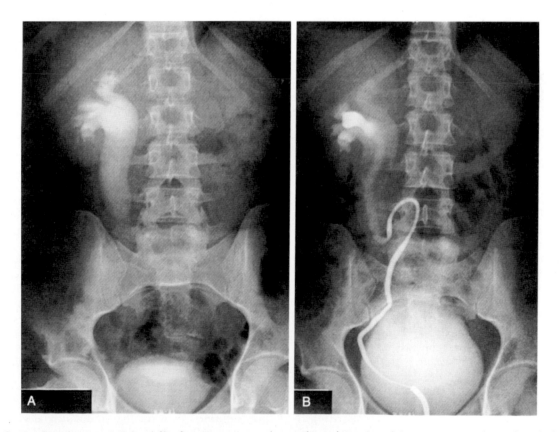

FIGURE 16–9. Circumcaval ureter. *A,* Delayed film from intravenous pyelogram shows obstruction of the upper ureter with significant hydronephrosis. *B,* Retrograde ureterogram shows the abnormal course of the ureter under the vena cava.

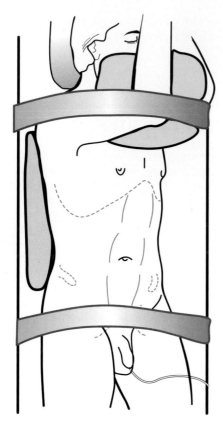

FIGURE 16–10. The patient is placed in a slight lateral position with a chest and buttocks roll placed.

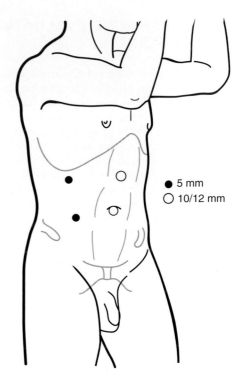

FIGURE 16–11. Three or four trocars are used with a 10-mm umbilical port for the camera. A 10-mm trocar is placed midway between the umbilicus and the xyphoid process, and a 5-mm trocar is lateral to the rectus in line with the umbilicus. An additional 5-mm trocar can be placed in the subcostal area for retraction as needed.

TROCAR PLACEMENT

Trocar placement follows a standard template. We use three 12-mm trocars. Locate the camera port at the umbilicus. Place the superior port in the midline approximately 10 cm superior to the umbilicus. Place the lateral port along the arcuate line approximately 10 cm lateral to the umbilicus (Fig. 16–11).

Step-by-Step Procedure

Using a Veress needle through the umbilicus, insufflate the abdominal cavity with CO_2 to 15 cm pressure. Make a 10-mm incision at the lateral port site. Use a Kelly clamp to spread the subcutaneous tissue off the fascial sheath. Using a Visiport with the 12-mm trocar and a 0-degree lens, enter the abdominal cavity. Place the two remaining ports at the appropriate positions under direct vision. Secure each trocar in place at the appropriate depth with a 2-0 silk stay suture.

Tilt the operating table 45 degrees toward the operating team to facilitate mobilization of the bowel. With the 30-degree lens, Maryland dissectors, and the suction-irrigator, move the bowel away from the lateral side wall to expose the white line of Toldt in its entirety. Then incise the white line with EndoShears using a combination of sharp dissection and electrocautery beginning at the iliac vessels and extending superiorly to the hepatic flexure and then diagonally to the renal hilum (Fig. 16–12).

Identify the interface between mesenteric fat and retroperitoneal fat. Medially mobilize the bowel and its mesentery to expose the interface between Gerota's fascia and the psoas muscle (Fig. 16–13). Then elevate Gerota's fascia off the psoas. Isolate the gonadal vein and drop it onto the psoas. Develop the interface between Gerota's fascia and the psoas, knowing that the ureter will begin to course medially and over the vena cava. Once this level is reached, drop Gerota's fascia and carry a more superficial dissection toward the renal hilum. Take great care at this level to sharply release the duodenum from the plane of dissection (Fig. 16–14). Once this is accomplished, the vena cava is readily visible. Identify the dilated renal pelvis and proximal ureter by their emergence from under the renal vein and their medially directed course (Fig. 16–15).

With the distal ureter dissected free of the anterior surface of the vena cava and the proximal ureter mobilized to the greatest extent possible from the medial and posterior vena cava, shift attention to planning for the reconstruction. It is critical to assess the length of the ureter. It is quite unlikely that dividing the ureter in one location will be adequate. More likely, divide the ureter in two locations, leaving the intervening posterior vena caval segment in situ. It is quite important to maintain adequate length to allow for an end-to-end spatulated repair. In addition, given that a ureteral stent is in place, it is critical to not cut or nick the stent during division of the ureter. Retract the stent from the renal pelvis rather than the urinary bladder.

After advancing the stent back into the renal pelvis, we perform our anastomosis. The anastomosis is done with free suturing or with the EndoStitch device using two running stitches, one for the posterior wall and one for the

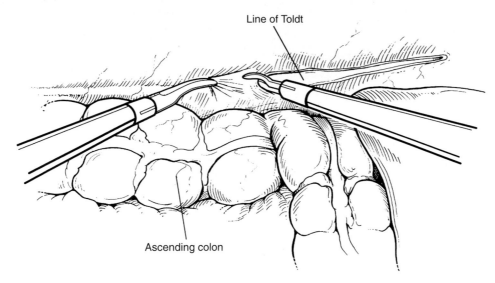

FIGURE 16–12. On the right side, the line of Toldt is sharply incised. Once the peritoneum has been opened, the colon can be reflected medially.

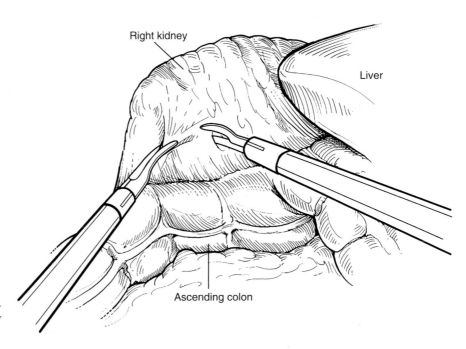

FIGURE 16–13. Renocolic attachments can be identified by medial traction on the colon and are sharply divided.

anterior wall. Place one clip using a Lapra-Ty absorbable suture clip applier (Ethicon, Cincinnati, OH) at the end of the suture to avoid the need for intracorporeal knot tying (Fig. 16–16).

Once the anastomosis is complete, place a Jackson-Pratt drain in the right upper quadrant, desufflate the abdomen, remove the trocars, and close the fascial defects.

POSTOPERATIVE MANAGEMENT

Postoperatively, patients are allowed clear liquids that are advanced to a regular diet as tolerated. For pain management, they are given morphine-based patient-controlled analgesia. Pain management is transitioned to oral narcotics the afternoon of postoperative day 1. The Foley catheter is typically removed

the morning of postoperative day 2. If the Jackson-Pratt drain output remains low and unchanged for the immediate 8 hours after Foley catheter removal, then it is also removed. Most patients are ready for discharge to home the afternoon of postoperative day 2.

The ureteral stent remains in place for 4 to 6 weeks postoperatively. The stent can be removed in the clinic. Patients are usually followed with laboratory tests and imaging 1 to 2 weeks after the removal of the stent and then on a 6-month basis for 2 years.

COMPLICATIONS

The general complications that can occur with all laparoscopic procedures are discussed elsewhere.

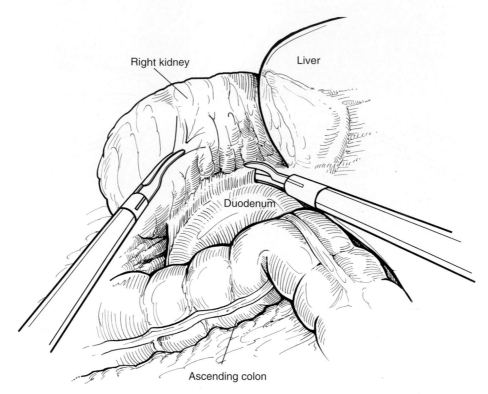

FIGURE 16–14. When the duodenum is found to obstruct the view of the renal pelvis and ureter, a Kocher maneuver is performed to complete mobilization of the bowel, exposing the inferior vena cava.

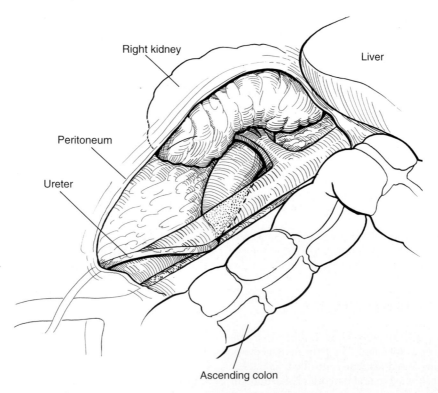

FIGURE 16–15. The lower pole of the kidney is located and elevated with a grasper, while the pelvis and ureter are identified and followed to the inferior vena cava.

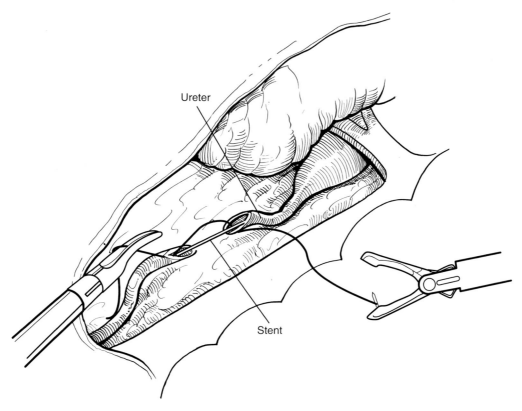

Ureter

Stent

FIGURE 16–16. The ureter is mobilized and divided. The free ends of the distal ureter are dissected from the inferior vena cava and spatulated. A 4-0 absorbable suture is used to approximate the ureter. Redundant ureter or pelvis can be excised as needed.

Long-term complication is limited to ureteral stricture. Stricture is a direct result of surgical technique. Management of this situation is discussed in detail elsewhere.

SPECIAL INSTRUMENTS

We use a standard laparoscopic tray for this procedure. In that tray are 5-mm instruments: two Maryland dissectors, a short- and long-tip right angle, EndoShears, a suction-irrigator, and an EndoStitch device.

Tips and Tricks

- Use a long ureteral stent to reduce the chance of advancing the distal curl out of the bladder and into the distal ureter.
- Use a LapraTy to fix the ends of sutures. This avoids the need for intracorporeal knot tying.
- Avoid the temptation to retrieve the posterior caval ureter. The inadvertent avulsion of a lumbar vein will quickly require conversion to open surgery.

REFERENCES

1. van Bommel E: Retroperitoneal fibrosis. Neth J Med 60(6):231–242, 2002.
2. Kavoussi LR, Clayman RV, Brunt LM, et al: Laparoscopic ureterolysis. J Urol 147(2):426–429, 1992.
3. Penalver C, Sanchez A, Charneco A, et al: Surgery for idiopathic retroperitoneal fibrosis by ureterolysis and ureteric protection with posterior pre-peritoneal fat flap. BJU 89:783–786, 2002.
4. Matsuda T, Arai Y, Muguruma K, et al: Laparoscopic ureterolysis for idiopathic retroperitoneal fibrosis. Eur Urol 26(4):286–290, 1994.
5. Boeckmann W, Wolff JM, Adam G, et al: Laparoscopic bilateral ureterolysis in Ormond's disease. Urol Int 56(2):133–136, 1996.
6. Puppo P, Carmignani G, Gallucci M, et al: Bilateral laparoscopic ureterolysis. Eur Urol 25(1):82–84, 1994.
7. Margossian H, Falcone T, Walters MD, et al: Laparoscopic repair of ureteral injuries. J Am Assoc Gynecol Laparosc 10(3):373–377, 2003.
8. Kumar M, Kumar R, Hemal AK, et al: Complications of retroperitoneoscopic surgery at one centre. BJU Int 87(7):607–612, 2001.
9. Baba S, Oya M, Miyahara M, et al: Laparoscopic surgical correction of circumcaval ureter. Urology 44(1):122–126, 1994.
10. Ishitoya S, Okubo K, Arai Y: Laparoscopic ureterolysis for retrocaval ureter. Br J Urol 77(1):162–163, 1996.
11. Matsuda T, Yasumoto R, Tsujino T: Laparoscopic treatment of a retrocaval ureter. Eur Urol 29(1):115–118, 1996.
12. Mugiya S, Suzuki K, Ohhira T, et al: Retroperitoneoscopic treatment of a retrocaval ureter. Int J Urol 6(8):419–422, 1999.
13. Salomon L, Hoznek A, Balian C, et al: Retroperitoneal laparoscopy of a retrocaval ureter. BJU Int 84(1):181–182, 1999.
14. Ameda K, Kakizaki H, Harabayashi T, et al: Laparsocopic ureteroureterostomy for retrocaval ureter. Int J Urol 8(2):71–74, 2001.
15. Miyazato M, Kimura T, Ohyama C, et al: Retroperitoneoscopic ureteroureterostomy for retrocaval ureter. Hinyokika Kiyo 48(1):25–28, 2002.
16. Bhandarkar DS, Lalmalani JG, Shivde S: Laparoscopic ureterolysis and reconstruction of a retrocaval ureter. Surg Endosc 17(11):1851–1852, 2003.
17. Ramalingam M, Selvarajan K: Laparoscopic transperitoneal repair of retrocaval ureter: Report of two cases. J Endourol 17(2):85–87, 2003.

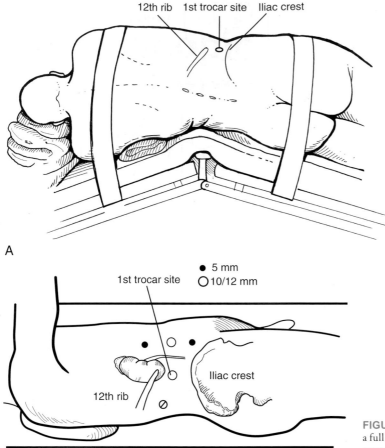

FIGURE 17–3. *A,* In the retroperitoneal approach, the patient is placed in a full lateral position. *B,* Trocar configuration for right-sided retroperitoneal access. The first trocar site is approximately 2 fingerbreadths below the 12th rib. Additional trocars are placed as needed for dissection and retraction.

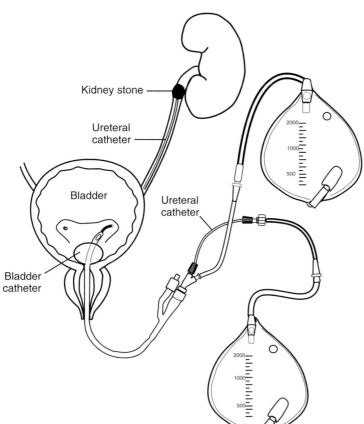

FIGURE 17–4. If a stent or catheter cannot be passed above the level of the stone, an open-ended catheter should be advanced to the stone. A Council Tip bladder catheter can be placed over the open-ended catheter and inflated in the bladder. Using a "Y" adapter attached to the bladder catheter, urine drainage can be achieved and a wire manipulated through the open-ended catheter once the stone has been removed.

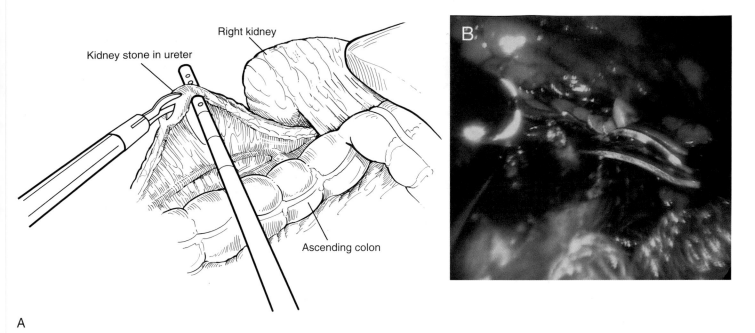

FIGURE 17–5. *A,* Once the stone is located in the ureter, the ureter is opened with laparoscopic scissors or a laparoscopic cold knife. *B,* The stone can usually be felt with the tip of the scissors.

Transperitoneal Approach

Medially reflect the colon over the stone, and expose the retroperitoneum. Using sharp and blunt dissection, expose the ureter while passing over the psoas muscle or crossing the iliac vessels. Isolate the ureter, and pass a vessel loop underneath it to tent it up and to prevent the stone from migrating. Alternatively, use a Babcock forceps to grasp the dilated ureter proximal to the uppermost calculus for the same reason. Usually, it is easy to identify the stone because its size causes the ureter to bulge adequately or because the graspers can palpate it. Using a cold knife, incise the ureter over the calculus beginning about 0.5 cm proximal to the stone (Fig. 17–5). Loosen the stone and lever it out with the help of a dissector (Fig. 17–6). Once the stone is extracted, use spoon forceps to remove the stone from the abdomen. Place stones that are too large to pass through the 10-mm port in a small laparoscopy bag and remove them at the conclusion of the procedure. Flush the ureter with saline to remove any stone fragments and to confirm patency. Leave the ureterotomy open if it is smaller than 1 cm or close it with interrupted 3-0 absorbable sutures (Fig. 17–7). Usually, if a stent is not already in place, do place a double-J stent either with the help of flexible cystoscopy or with laparoscopic manipulation introducing the double-J through one of the laparoscopic ports. A stent is not always needed unless the ureteral incision is not sutured. Always leave a drain in the retroperitoneal space. Following fluoroscopy to confirm a stone-free status and proper stent placement, remove ports after CO_2 deflation.

Retroperitoneal Approach

After placing the trocars, the steps are the same as in the transperitoneal approach. Postoperative management is also the same.

POSTOPERATIVE MANAGEMENT

The patient resumes oral food intake on postoperative day 1, the Foley catheter is removed on postoperative day 2, and the drain is removed the same afternoon if the output is less than 30 mL. The stent is removed 4 weeks postoperatively, and an intravenous pyelogram is performed 6 weeks later. Further follow-up varies.

COMPLICATIONS

Complications were minor and mainly constituted short-term postoperative fever, ileus, deep venous thrombosis, incisional hernias, subcutaneous emphysema, and subcutaneous hematomas. Urinary leak was commonly seen,[7] but eventually tapered off. Harewood and associates[10] reported a urinary leak in 55.5%, but this was of 3-day duration only. Keeley and colleagues[11] and Skrepetis and associates[8] reported longer leakages of 12 and 10 days, respectively, which were treated conservatively. They were attributed to the fact that no internal stents were placed. A urinoma requiring drainage was reported by Micali and colleagues,[12] but in this case no drain was placed. Bowel and vascular injuries and injuries of neighboring organs are always a risk during laparoscopic surgery, although they were not reported in these series of procedures.

There are no long-term results concerning the incidence of ureteral stricture postoperatively. In most cases, the ureterotomy was made with a cold knife because the use of scissors to cut a frequently thick ureter can be tedious. Some authors used the diathermy hook[10] or a neodymium:YAG laser,[3] but no data are reported about the incidence of postoperative ureteral stenosis in this setting.

CHAPTER 18

Laparoscopic Ureteral Reimplantation and Boari Flap

Koon Ho Rha

In the past decade, laparoscopy has been successfully used for both the obliterative and reconstructive management of urologic disease. We have seen not only an advance in the technology available to perform these procedures but also an effort on the part of laparoscopic urologists to refine their techniques to allow them to perform more complicated procedures.

INDICATIONS AND CONTRAINDICATIONS

There are various indications for ureteral reimplantation in adults. For adults with injury or obstruction affecting the distal 3 to 4 cm of the ureter, such as stricture, penetrating trauma, or intraoperative injury, perform a ureteral reimplantation with a psoas hitch or Boari flap. Perform direct ureteral reimplantation if a tension-free anastomosis is possible; otherwise, use a psoas hitch or Boari flap. Perform a direct, nontunneled anastomosis if postoperative reflux is not an issue; otherwise, create a submucosal tunnel. Use a double-J stent postoperatively if desired, and place drains.

The psoas hitch is an effective means to bridge a defect of the lower third of the ureter. Indications include distal ureteral injury, ureteral fistulas secondary to pelvic surgery, segmental resection of a distal ureteral tumor, and failed ureteral reimplantation.[1] Ureteral defects proximal to the pelvic brim usually require more than a simple psoas hitch alone. A psoas hitch can provide an additional 5 cm of length compared with ureteral reimplantation alone. Its advantages over a Boari flap include simplicity, improved vascularity, ease of endoscopic surveillance, and minimal voiding difficulties.

Mid ureteral defects present a particular surgical challenge because this area has a tenuous blood supply and there are potential problems achieving a tension-free repair. When the diseased segment is too long or ureteral mobility too limited to perform a primary ureteral reimplantation, a Boari flap may be a useful alternative. A Boari flap can be constructed to comfortably bridge a 10- to 15-cm defect, and spiraled bladder flaps can reach to the renal pelvis in some circumstances. As with a psoas hitch, preoperatively completely visualize the ureter and evaluate bladder function. Preoperatively address bladder outlet obstruction and neurogenic dysfunction, and realize that a small bladder capacity predicts difficulty.

Although the ureteral reimplantation, psoas hitch, and Boari flap have conventionally been performed by open surgery, the advantages of the laparoscopic technique have rapidly come into the limelight. Shorter hospital stay, rapid recovery, less postoperative pain, and better cosmesis are the main advantages of laparoscopic surgery. The success of every laparoscopic procedure depends on proper patient selection and the surgeon's skill and confidence with laparoscopy.

Improvements in the skills of laparoscopic urologists and the advent of instruments to facilitate suturing (e.g., Lapra-Ty [Ethicon, Cincinnati, OH], clips to replace intracorporeal knotting, and advances in staple and clip technology) have facilitated a renewed interest in laparoscopic reconstructive surgery of the lower urinary tract. The latest development in reconstructive laparoscopic urology has been the advent of the semiautomatic suturing device, the EndoStitch (Auto Suture, U.S. Surgical, Norwalk, CT). With this device, the needle and suture can be rapidly passed through both edges of the tissue without the surgeon needing to physically grasp the needle. This greatly speeds up the sewing process; indeed, in one clinical series of pyeloplasty, Moore and associates[2] estimated that the introduction of the EndoStitch into their procedures reduced the operating room time by 2.1 hours. At present, almost all types of urologic open reconstructive procedures have been accomplished laparoscopically: urinary diversion, bladder reconstruction, ureteral reimplantation, and urethrovesical anastomosis following radical prostatectomy. This chapter reviews the development of ureteral reimplantation and Boari flap.

PATIENT PREOPERATIVE EVALUATION AND PREPARATION

Preoperatively, measure the length of defective ureter on antegrade and retrograde radiographs. Note that the length usually is over or underestimated; it is rarely accurate. After thoroughly reviewing all options, including psoas hitch and other endoscopic methods, if the laparoscopic Boari flap is selected, evaluate the bladder volume carefully. Review previous radiation or previous injury to the bladder. Carefully review previous pelvic surgeries to reveal additional information.

OPERATING ROOM CONFIGURATION AND PATIENT POSITIONING

Patient positioning is the same for all of the ureteral reimplantation procedures. As with other laparoscopic procedures, the operating room is configured so that the entire team can view the procedure on the monitor. Position the patient in a supine position, and carefully secure the patient to the table so that an

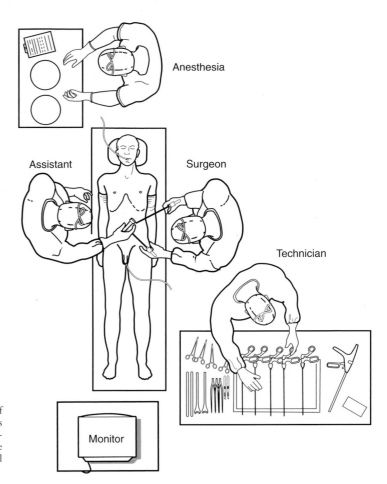

FIGURE 18–1. The operating room is configured so that the entire staff can view the procedure. The patient is positioned supine with the arms tucked. Several bands of tape are used to secure the patient at the shoulders, hips, and legs. The patient needs to be carefully secured to the table to allow being placed in the head-down position to allow bowel to fall away from the pelvis, improving exposure to the bladder.

exaggerated head-down position can be used to move the bowel contents away from the bladder (Fig. 18–1).

Assess the length and location of the ureteral stricture by preoperative antegrade and retrograde studies. With the patient under general anesthesia, prepare the abdomen and genitalia in the operative field. Place an orogastric tube and have the Foley catheter within the field to allow access during the procedure. Achieve pneumoperitoneum using a Veress needle.

TROCAR PLACEMENT

Insert the initial trocar at the umbilicus using Veress access with a 10/12-mm supraumbilical port for the camera. Place two additional 5-mm working trocars under direct vision at the level of the iliac crest along the lateral edge of the rectus muscle, triangulating these with the camera port. These ports are used for the initial colonic dissection (Fig. 18–2). In female patients, make the initial dissection in the peritoneal fold between the bladder and uterus to gain access to the ureters in the region of the trigone. In male patients, the ureter can be seen as it crosses posterior to the vas deferens. Create a peritoneal window, and free and elevate the ureter inferior to the vas deferens. Mobilize each ureter once it can be elevated onto the base of the bladder sufficiently for placement in a detrusor tunnel. Dissect the ureter up to the juxtavesical region and transect it after ligation of the distal end. Then spatulate the ureter; this is usually easily performed because the proximal ureter is dilated and accommodates the scissors without difficulty.

Anteriorly mobilize the bladder to develop the prevesical space. Similarly, posteriorly dissect the bladder to maximize mobility before opening it. Choose the site of the ureteral reimplantation so that it is as inferior and medial as possible. Fill the bladder with 150 to 200 mL of saline. Using the scissors, hook, and needle-tip electrode, incise the detrusor about 3 cm, allowing the mucosa to bulge out between the muscularis edges. Be careful not to enter the mucosa before being ready to make the anastomosis because the bladder will rapidly decompress, making further dissection of the muscularis difficult.

Open the mucosa in the most distal portion of the incision. Take the first stitch through the apex of the spatulated ureter and the proximal end of the hole in the mucosa using a 3-0 absorbable suture on a round-body needle following an intracorporeal suturing technique. Make eight interrupted sutures. This fixes the ureter in the detrusor groove created earlier. Before taking the last few stitches, place the double-J stent. Then close the detrusor with three interrupted sutures of 3-0 polyglycolic acid to make the submucosal tunnel.

Laparoscopic Ureteral Reimplantation

McDougall and colleagues[3] described ureteral reimplantation into the bladder in 1995. They used the Lich-Gregoir technique. They used intracorporeal suturing technique to perform the ureteral-vesical anastomosis over which the detrusor tunnel was closed, by 3-0 polyglactin suture in four pigs and with tacking staples in three pigs.

Ehrlich and associates[4] successfully treated vesicoureteral reflux in two children using the laparoscopic technique. The operative time was 2 to 3 hours. In both cases, they performed an extravesical and Lich-Gregoir repair. There were no complications. Two-month follow-up showed no reflux or hydronephrosis. Reddy and Evans[5] first performed a laparoscopic ureteroneocystostomy on a 74-year-old patient who presented with hydronephrosis after transurethral resection of the prostate and cystoscopy revealed an obliterated left ureteral orifice. They laparoscopically transected the dilated ureter and advanced the nephroureteral catheter into the bladder through a neocystotomy. The ureteroneocystostomy was completed with six 3-0 polyglactin interrupted sutures. The operative time was 4.5 hours, and at 3 weeks postoperatively the ureter was patent with no extravasation.

Yohannes and associates[6] described the technique in detail, reporting their experience in a case of lower-ureteral stricture. They used an EndoStitch device to assist with the suturing. Yohannes and colleagues[7] later described robot-assisted laparoscopic reimplantation, but it was a simple ureterovesical refluxing anastomosis.

The main indication for ureteroneocystostomy in children is vesicoureteral reflux, and the ureteral dissection in the perivesical region is easy because the planes are virgin and untouched. In the adults, however, one indication for ureteroneocystostomy is iatrogenic injury of the ureter, and posthysterectomy injury is a common indication. Consequently, the dissection of the distal ureter can be extremely difficult, and the degree of mobilization of the ureter may be limited. In addition, because the level of the ureteral injury is not certain, it may be necessary to tackle higher levels of injury, and it may be necessary to manage with lesser lengths of ureter. This, in turn, means that the surgeon must be ready for more difficult surgical steps such as the psoas hitch and full mobilization of the ureter. It is imperative in the child that the detrusorrhaphy achieve a secure antireflux mechanism, whereas in the adult, the antireflux repair generally is not considered important. This is probably because the procedure becomes more complicated and because of fear that the detrusorrhaphy will cause an element of vesicoureteral obstruction.

Psoas Hitch

If the anastomosis is on tension, a psoas hitch can be performed. The psoas muscle is already exposed by the earlier dissection of the ureter. Use polypropylene 2-0 on a round-body needle. Make the first pass into the bladder muscle lateral to the neoureterocystostomy site. Then pass the needle into the psoas muscle, taking care not to injure any other structure. Make a knot with help from the assistant, who uses the fourth port, to prevent the knot from slipping. Take a second suture lateral to the first that supports the hitch. Perform the psoas hitch after the ureterovesical anastomosis, based on the open surgical technique described by Hendren.[8]

After the repair is complete, remove instruments and trocars after checking for bleeding and visceral injury. Close the fascial defects and skin of each port with absorbable sutures. Leave a bladder catheter in place for several days.

Laparoscopic Boari Flap

The Boari flap is a viable alternative for ureteral reconstruction when long defects of the mid to lower ureter must be bridged to the bladder. In 1894, Casati and Boari[9] first described this technique in a canine model, and in 1947 it was first applied in humans.[10] Fergany and associates[11] described a laparoscopic Boari flap in a porcine model. Fugita and colleagues[12] described three cases of the laparoscopic Boari flap technique for lower-ureteral stricture. Excellent outcomes were achieved in their patients with regard to symptomatic relief, radiologic results, and renal function. In 2005, Castillo and associates[13] also described eight cases of the laparoscopic Boari flap and expressed that the laparoscopic Boari flap was a feasible alternative surgical technique in patients with long distal ureteral strictures.

PROCEDURE

With the patient under general anesthesia, prepare the abdomen and genitalia into the operative field. Pass a Foley catheter, and place the patient supine. Use a Veress needle to achieve pneumoperitoneum. Place two 10/12-mm ports, including one through the umbilical incision for the camera and one at McBurney's point under direct vision. Place a 5-mm port in the lateral edge of the rectus muscle at the level of the umbilicus under direct vision.

Reflect the colon medially by incising the line of Toldt from the liver on the right and spleen on the left sides to the medial umbilical ligament. At this point, extend the incision medial to the umbilical ligament on the anterior abdominal wall. The ureter is then visible above the level of iliac vessels and freed as distally as possible. It is always important to preserve the periureteral tissue during its dissection to avoid ureteral devascularization. Transect normal ureter above the stricture area and spatulate it posteriorly on the normal ureter proximal end (Fig. 18–3).

Fill the bladder with 150 to 200 mL of saline, and incise the overlying anterior and contralateral peritoneum. Ligate and transect the urachus with clips. With blunt dissection, free the

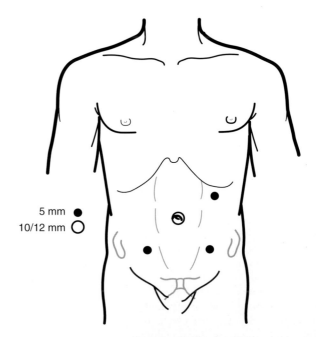

5 mm ●
10/12 mm ○

FIGURE 18–2. After insufflation with the Veress needle, the trocars are placed. A 10/12-mm trocar is placed at the umbilicus for the camera. Two additional trocars are placed at the level of the anterior superior iliac crest lateral to the rectus muscles.

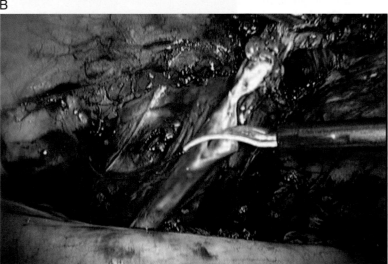

Ureter

Bladder

Ureter
stricture

A

B

C

FI
inc

bl.
su
(E
sa

2
bl.
as
fla
be
2-
an
an
Af
st
ro
th
th
th
po

FIGURE 18–3. *A,* A peritoneal window is created and the ureter identified. It can be difficult to locate the precise area of ureteral stricture. An opened catheter can be advanced to the level of the stricture during the case with a flexible scope in the male patient or at the start of the procedure in a female patient. *B,* Once the stricture is identified, the ureter is incised. *C,* It is helpful to spatulate the ureter before complete transection.

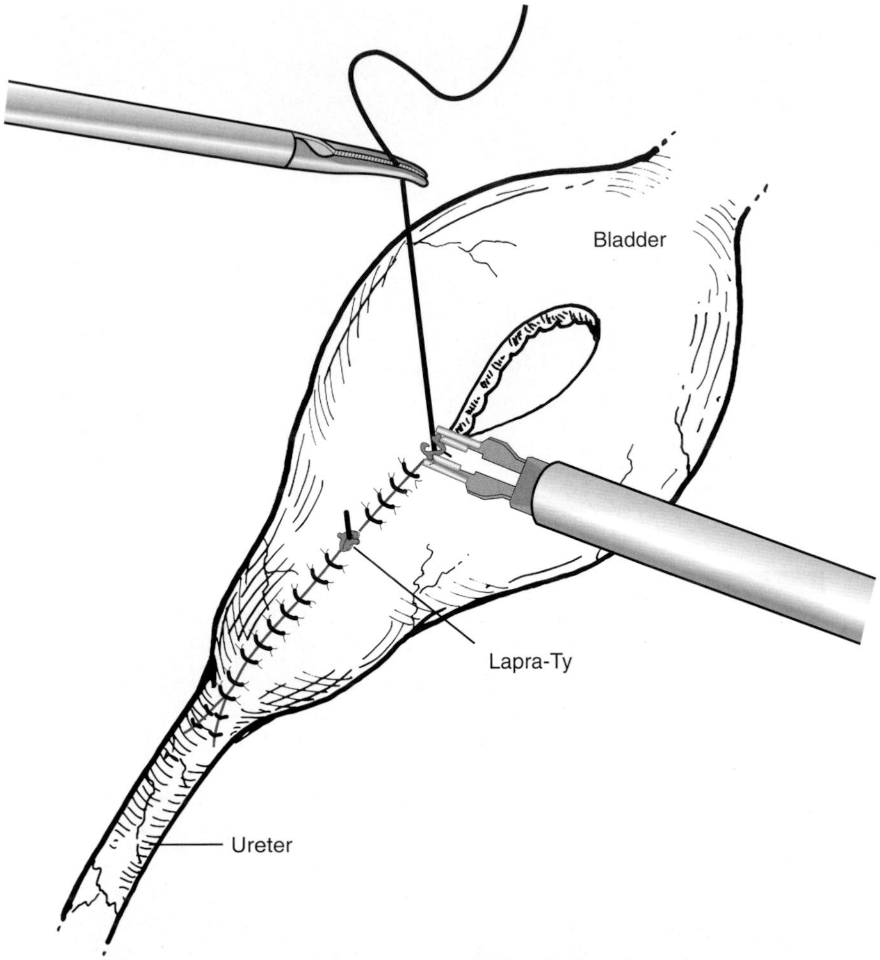

Bladder

Lapra-Ty

Ureter

A

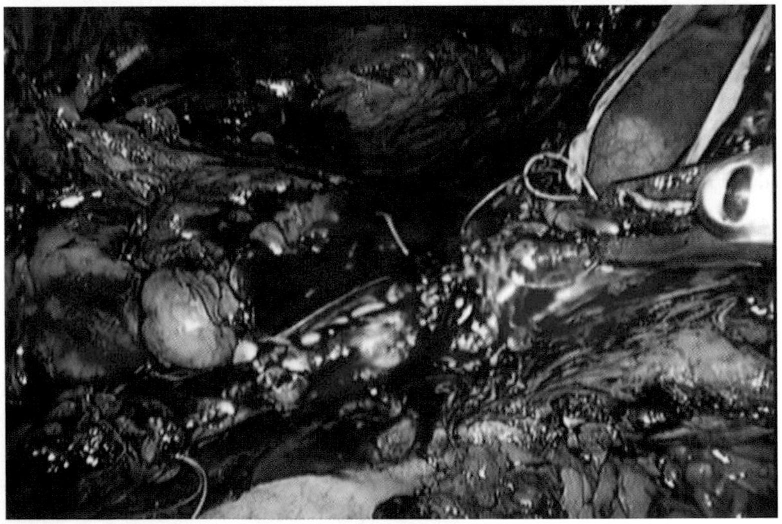

B

FIGURE 18–8. *A,* The Lapra-Ty (Ethicon) is useful when closing a long suture line, because shorter sutures are usually easier to work with during laparoscopy. *B,* The Lapra-Ty is being applied to the first suture closing the bladder.

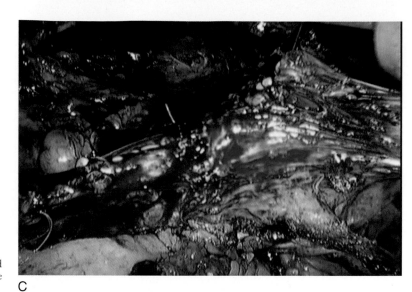

FIGURE 18–8, cont'd. *C,* The anastomosis is complete, and the last tie can be substituted with a Lapra-Ty, making the suture line watertight.

C

Radiologically follow the patients every 3 to 6 months for any obstructions after repair.

COMPLICATIONS

Prolonged urinary drainage through the drain may occur. If the ureteral stent or catheter is well placed, the condition is usually temporary. Review the surgical repair and suturing of the flap, and confirm the position of the ureteral stent or catheter. Urinary obstruction after removal of stent may occur. Diuretic renogram is helpful in determining actual obstruction. If the obstruction is present, balloon dilation of ureteral narrowing may relieve the obstruction.

Urinary frequency and other voiding symptoms due to the reduced bladder capacity are common in the immediate postoperative period. Usually, the bladder capacity increases gradually and the frequency does not persist to the same degree.

SUMMARY

Laparoscopic ureteral reimplantation, psoas hitch, and Boari flap are feasible surgical techniques in patients with distal ureteral stricture or long mid and distal ureteral stricture. Medium-term follow-up demonstrates symptomatic renal function and radiographic outcomes similar to those of open technique. Advanced laparoscopic skills are definitely needed to perform this procedure. Currently and in the near future, this procedure will be widely performed with robot-assisted laparoscopy technique.[14]

REFERENCES

1. Rodo Salas J, Martin Hortiguela E, Salarich de Arbell J: [Psoas fixation of the bladder. An efficient aid in case of repeat surgery of the uretero-vesical junction] [in Spanish]. Arch Esp Urol 44:125, 1991.
2. Moore RG, Averch TD, Schulam PG, et al: Laparoscopic pyeloplasty: Experience with the initial 30 cases. J Urol 157:459–462, 1997.
3. McDougall EM, Urban DA, Kerbl K, et al: Laparoscopic repair of vesicoureteral reflux utilizing the Lich-Gregoir technique in the pig model. J Urol 153:497–500, 1995.
4. Ehrlich RM, Gershman A, Fuchs G: Laparoscopic vesicoureteroplasty in children: Initial case reports. Urology 43:255–262, 1994.
5. Reddy PK, Evans RM: Laparoscopic ureteroneocystostomy. J Urol 152:2057–2060, 1994.
6. Yohannes P, Gershbaum D, Rotariu PE: Management of ureteral stricture disease during laparoscopic ureteroneocystostomy. J Endourol 15:839–843, 2001.
7. Yohannes P, Chiou PK, Pelinkovic D: Pure robot-assisted laparoscopic ureteral reimplantation for ureteral stricture disease: Case report. J Endourol 17:891–893, 2003.
8. Hendren WH: Urinary undiversion: Refunctionalization of the previously diverted urinary tract. In Campbell's Urology, 6th ed. Philadelphia, WB Saunders, 1992, pp 2721–2749.
9. Casati E, Boari A: Contributo sperimentale alla plastica dell'uretere. Comunicazione preventive. Atti Acad Sci Med Nat 14(3):149, 1894.
10. Ockerblad NF: Reimplantation of the ureter into the bladder by a flap method. J Urol 57:845, 1947.
11. Fergany A, Gill IS, Abdel-Samee A, et al: Laparoscopic bladder flap ureteral reimplantation: Survival porcine study. J Urol 166:1920, 2001.
12. Fugita OE, Dinlenc C, Kavoussi L: The laparoscopic Boari flap. J Urol 166:51–53, 2001.
13. Castillo OA, Litvak JP, Kerkebe M, et al: Early experience with the laparoscopic Boari flap at a single institution. J Urol 173:862–865, 2005.
14. Yohannes P, Chiou RK, Pelinkovic D: Pure robot-assisted laparoscopic ureteral reimplantation for ureteral stricture disease: Case report. J Endourol 17:891–893, 2003.

CHAPTER 19

Laparoscopic Adrenalectomy

Blake D. Hamilton

Since the initial report of laparoscopic adrenalectomy in 1992,[1] this procedure has become the gold standard for the removal of most adrenal pathology. Now there is little debate regarding the merits of this technique. Curiously, there has never been a prospective randomized study comparing open and laparoscopic adrenalectomy, yet in the published literature, there are more than 400 entries from around the world describing the surgical experience with laparoscopic adrenalectomy. At this point, the jury has weighed in so favorably on the side of laparoscopy that a randomized trial will likely never be done.[2–9]

Rather, discussion now centers on questions such as which laparoscopic approach is best? What about adrenal sparing with partial excision? How large is too large for a laparoscopic approach? Is this technique ever appropriate for malignant disease? In this chapter, I describe the current techniques for transperitoneal and retroperitoneal adrenalectomy. I also address the current indications for laparoscopic adrenalectomy and try to answer the above questions. What is clear is that laparoscopic adrenalectomy has become the standard for adrenal surgery. For additional perspective on this procedure, several excellent reviews have been published.[10–12]

INDICATIONS AND CONTRAINDICATIONS

Laparoscopic adrenalectomy is clearly preferred for benign adrenal tumors. These tumors can be classified as functional or nonfunctional (Table 19–1). A *nonfunctional* adrenal tumor generally manifests as an incidental finding on computed tomography or magnetic resonance imaging studies obtained for other purposes. The justification for the removal of a nonfunctional tumor lies in the size of the adrenal mass; a lesion that is large (>5 cm) at diagnosis or is shown to be enlarging on serial examinations has a greater possibility of being malignant.

Metastatic lesions from nonadrenal primary tumors are included in the nonfunctional category. Most commonly metastasizing from lung, breast, kidney, or skin (melanoma), these tumors may be indistinguishable from benign adenomas on preoperative images. If the tumor is a solitary metastasis, laparoscopic removal may be appropriate, although the benefit to the patient must be carefully considered. There are a few relatively small studies of such tumors in the literature.[13,14]

Functional adrenal tumors arise from the adrenal cortex or medulla and are manifested in a variety of ways (see Table 19–1). Because these tumors are relatively uncommon, their discovery is frequently delayed. The diagnosis and evaluation of these various pathologic states are beyond the scope of this chapter but can be found in standard texts on adrenal diseases.[15]

The perioperative treatment of the various disease states is a critical element in the management of affected patients and must not be neglected.

Excessive size is a relative contraindication to laparoscopic adrenalectomy, and there is debate regarding the upper limit of adrenal size amenable to the laparoscopic approach. Most authors would agree that 10- to 12-cm masses can be removed laparoscopically.[11] But patients must be carefully selected because these larger masses are technically more difficult to remove and have a greater likelihood of representing adrenocortical carcinoma. There are now several series of larger (>5 cm) adrenal masses that have been reported.[16–18] Such lesions are infrequent and should be undertaken by experienced laparoscopic surgeons.

Laparoscopic adrenalectomy for adrenal cortical carcinoma is controversial because a poor laparoscopic resection may be harmful to the patient. These malignant lesions are generally large and invasive. However, there are some reports of successful laparoscopic removal of malignant adrenal tumors.[13,14,19] Just as in open dissection, care must be taken to minimize manipulation of the adrenal tumor, obtain wide margins, and avoid tumor spillage.

Previous surgery may be a relative contraindication to laparoscopic adrenalectomy, in that extensive scarring may make the procedure more difficult. With the option of transperitoneal or retroperitoneal laparoscopic access, there is more flexibility in patients with previous surgery and these patients can often undergo a laparoscopic procedure.

PATIENT PREOPERATIVE EVALUATION AND PREPARATION

Preoperative counseling covers the standard risks of surgery, as well as the specific risks of injury to spleen or liver, kidney, and major vascular structures. Discuss the possibility of conversion to open surgery, including personal experience with the intended procedure. Most large series report a low conversion rate of 2% to 5%.[20,21] Administer broad-spectrum intravenous antibiotics at the outset of the procedure and continue them for 24 hours. After administration of general anesthesia, place a Foley catheter and orogastric tube.

Treat the patient who has pheochromocytoma for several weeks before surgery with an appropriate agent. I use phenoxybenzamine, a long-acting α-adrenergic blocker, but others have reported using selective α-blockers or calcium channel blockers. Consult with the anesthetist as part of preoperative planning. Give patients with glucocorticoid-producing tumors perioperative hydrocortisone. Because the contralateral adrenal

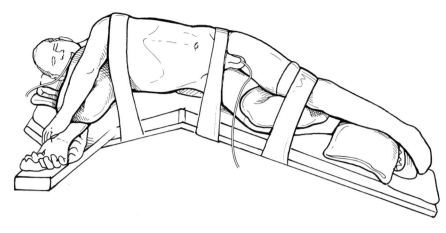

FIGURE 19–1. In the transperitoneal approach the patient is placed in the modified flank position. The flank is placed directly over the break in the table so that the table can be flexed. The arms are carefully padded and secured. Wide cloth tape is used to secure the hips and chest.

TABLE 19–1. INDICATIONS FOR LAPAROSCOPIC ADRENALECTOMY

Functional Adrenal Tumors
Aldosterone-secreting tumor (Conn's syndrome)
Cortisol-secreting tumor (Cushing's syndrome)
Virilizing tumor
Pheochromocytoma

Nonfunctional Adrenal Tumors
Incidental adrenal mass >5 cm
Adrenal mass <5 cm but enlarging on serial examinations
Solitary metastasis from nonadrenal primary (e.g., breast, lung, kidney, skin)

is severely suppressed by the excess function of the tumor, cortisol replacement is often necessary for weeks to months after surgery. Patients with aldosterone-secreting tumors need to undergo several weeks of adequate hypertension control and correction of hypokalemia.

OPERATING ROOM CONFIGURATION AND PATIENT POSITIONING

Transperitoneal Approach

For transperitoneal adrenalectomy, place the patient in a modified flank position, 20 to 30 degrees back from vertical (Fig. 19–1). Use a beanbag device or a padded roll to keep the patient in position, if needed. Do not flex the table, except in the event of conversion to open surgery, in which case the table is flexed as needed to improve exposure. Extend the lower arm on a standard arm board and place an axillary roll just caudad to the axilla. Bring the upper arm across the body and support it with a Krause (sling) rest, double arm board, or several pillows. Adequately extend the upper arm to avoid undue strain on the upper shoulder joint. Pad both arms under the elbows and wrists. Place sequential pneumatic compression devices on the legs, which are gently flexed with a pillow between them and foam under the feet and ankles. Place wide tape strips across the hips and chest to secure the patient to the table. Now laterally tilt the operating table to change body position during the procedure. Both surgeon and assistant stand on the patient's ventral side (Fig. 19–2). The technician stands at the patient's

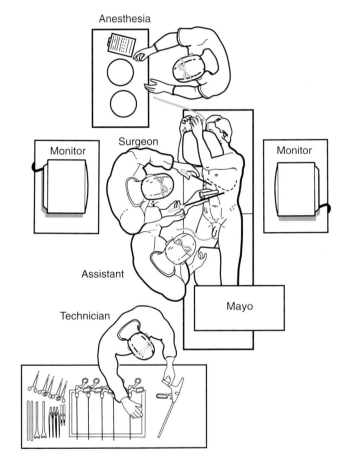

FIGURE 19–2. OR setup for the transperitoneal approach.

feet or on the opposite side, and two monitors are positioned so that all members of the surgical team can view the procedure.

Retroperitoneal Approach

Patient positioning in the retroperitoneal approach is similar to the transperitoneal approach except that the patient is in a full flank position (Fig. 19–3). Place the flank directly over the table break with the patient on a beanbag. Flexion of the table is recommended to open the space between the 12th rib and the iliac crest. With the table flexed, adjust the bed to create a level operating surface (usually by raising the head). Extend both

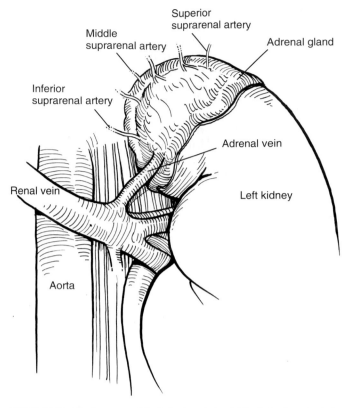

FIGURE 19–11. Anatomy of the left adrenal gland. The left adrenal vein is usually found medial to the level of insertion of the gonadal vein on the renal vein and at the lateral edge of the aorta. Practically speaking, the adrenal vein is usually more medial than expected.

arterial supply consists of an extensive array of small arteries around the medial side of the adrenal that can be easily handled with electrocautery or other dissecting energy (Fig. 19–13).

Once dissected entirely, place the adrenal into a retrieval bag and remove it through the largest port site (Fig. 19–14). Close the port sites in standard fashion (see Chapter 4).

Right-Sided Adrenalectomy

Carry the dissection down along the ascending colon and medially just below the liver until the colon falls away, exposing the kidney. There is often minimal or even no mobilization of the colon if the suprarenal fossa is easily exposed by lifting up the liver. Mobilize the liver from its abdominal wall attachments high up along its lateral aspect (Fig. 19–15). Retraction of the liver, which is necessary to sufficiently uncover the adrenal gland and complete the dissection, can be achieved with a retractor through either the most medial or most lateral port (Fig. 19–16).

The right adrenal gland is closer to the inferior vena cava (IVC) than the left adrenal is to the aorta, which makes this side trickier. The right adrenal vein usually arises from the posterolateral aspect of the IVC (Fig. 19–17). If the adrenal gland is readily identified, dissect right along the edge of the gland. I expose the IVC directly and extend this dissection up to the top of the adrenal gland. Just above the junction of the IVC and renal vein, use a blunt retractor to push the adrenal gland laterally, away from the IVC, creating a working space. Divide the vessels along the medial edge of the adrenal with electrocautery until the short adrenal vein is identified. At this point, expose the short adrenal vein with a right-angle dissector

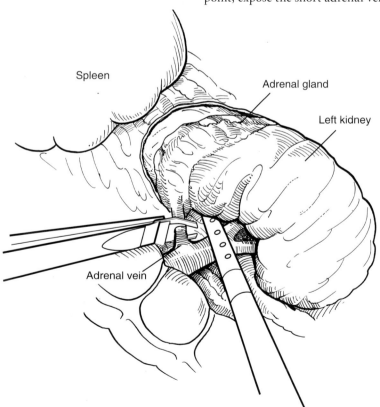

FIGURE 19–12. After the vein is ligated and divided, complete dissection is performed. This can be done by lifting or pushing the adrenal rather than grasping it. Electrocautery effectively divides the many small feeding vessels. The remainder of the dissection consists of freeing the adrenal from its bed. Infrequently, additional variant veins may require clips and should be identified.

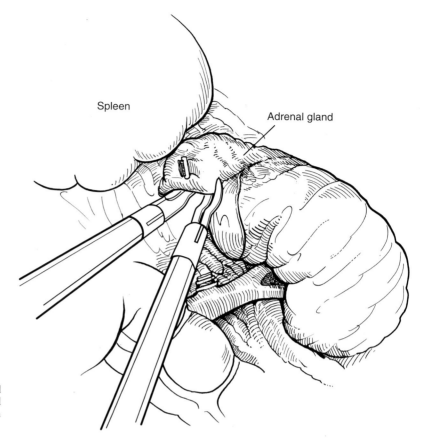

FIGURE 19–18. At the me
the short adrenal vein is i
right-angle dissector and di
there is adequate room divid
stapler.

FIGURE 19–13. Once the adrenal vein is divided, the adrenal gland is separated from the upper pole of the kidney and freed posteriorly, leaving the superior attachments, which are then divided with electrocautery or other energy.

FIGURE 19–19. With t
remainder of the dissection
small vessels feeding the ac
vein the adrenal is dissected
inferior attachments to the
released.

and divide it between c
(Fig. 19–18). Surgeon
with the vascular stap
space between the ven
in order to prevent avu
and activation of the s
additional venous bran
even the hepatic veins
during the dissection.
adrenal arteries with c

With the main adr
dissection is less worr
pletely free, place it in
port site. Close the in

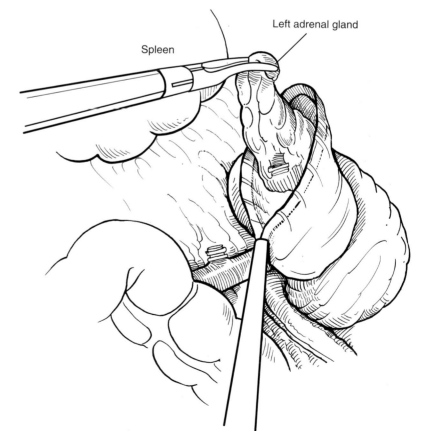

FIGURE 19–14. The dissected adrenal gland is placed into a commercial retrieval pouch and removed through the largest port site.

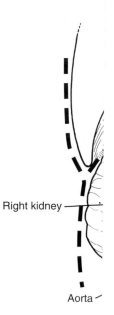

Right kidney —

Aorta ⌐

FIGURE 19–15.
peritoneum is open
liver until the colon
the liver is mobilize
lateral aspect, stayi
inferior vena cava.

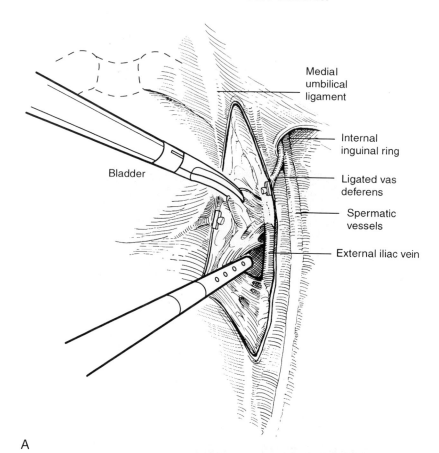

Medial umbilical ligament

Internal inguinal ring

Bladder

Ligated vas deferens

Spermatic vessels

External iliac vein

A

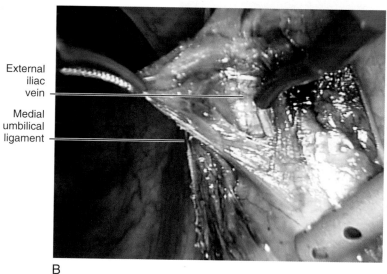

External iliac vein

Medial umbilical ligament

B

FIGURE 20–7. *A,* Gentle traction is used on the nodal packet and blunt dissection with the tip of the irrigator aspirator serially elevates tissue away from the external iliac vein to expose the anterior surface. *B,* The hook electrode can be used to divide attachments, small blood vessels, and small lymphatic channels. This plane of dissection is followed until the muscles of the pelvic side wall are encountered.

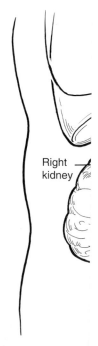

Right kidney

FIGURE 19–16.
the adrenal gland
fan retractor throu

In some settings (bladder, urethral, penile, and prostate cancer), an extended lymph node dissection to incorporate the common, internal, and external iliac lymph nodes as well might be performed.[6] Proceed in a manner similar to conventional node dissection, except the lateral border of dissection is along the common iliac artery up to the genitofemoral nerve. The medial extent of dissection is the medial border of the bladder and ureter. The dissection caudally remains the same as the modified or standard lymph node dissection, but cranially the dissection is carried above the common iliac artery bifurcation.

POSTOPERATIVE MANAGEMENT

Postoperatively, patient management is dictated by the additional procedures that are performed at the time of node dissection. Patients undergoing a node dissection only are routinely discharged on the day following surgery after showing that they can tolerate a regular diet. In patients undergoing additional simultaneous procedures such as laparoscopic radical prostatectomy, the postoperative course is determined by the additional

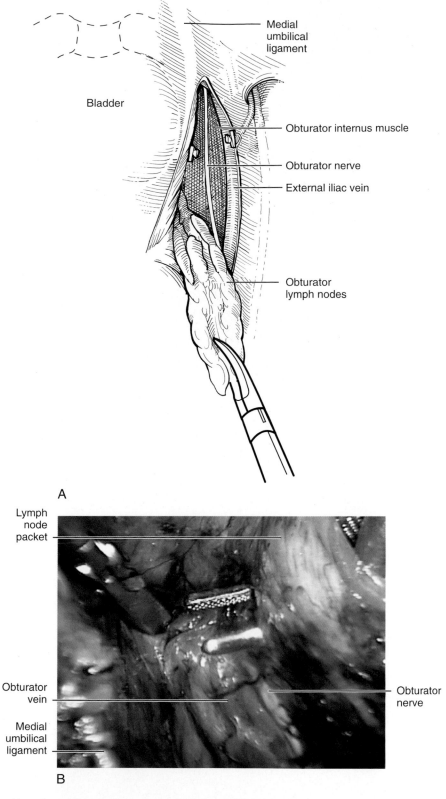

Medial umbilical ligament

Bladder

Obturator internus muscle

Obturator nerve

External iliac vein

Obturator lymph nodes

A

Lymph node packet

Obturator vein

Medial umbilical ligament

Obturator nerve

B

FIGURE 20–8. *A,* The lateral boundary of the node dissection is extended caudally until the pubic bone is reached. At this level, a 10-mm right angle is placed around the nodal packet just caudal to the node of Cloquet. *B,* After securing the distal lymphatic pedicle between clips, it is then transected with scissors.

Continued

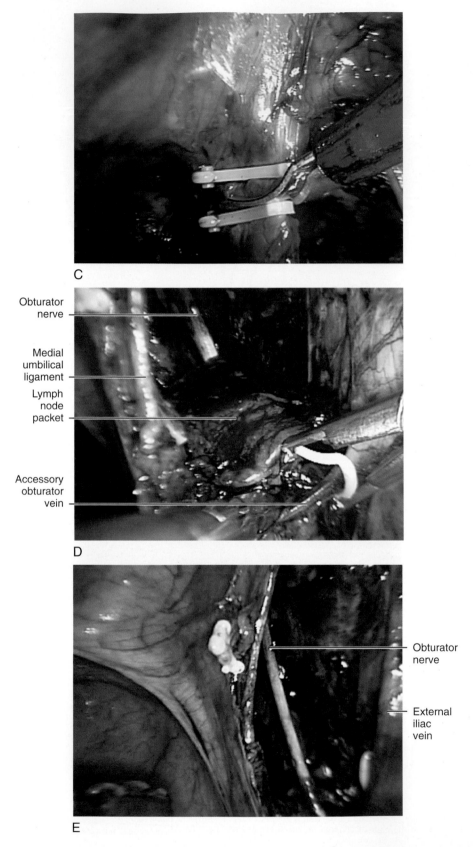

FIGURE 20–8, cont'd. *C,* During dissection of the nodal packet, an accessory obturator vein is often identified joining the medial side of the external iliac vein. Transection between clips simplifies removal of the node packet. *D,* The cephalad extent of the node packet is transected at the level of the bifurcation of the iliac vessels. *E,* Careful inspection of the obturator fossa ensures that all nodal tissue has been removed and that there is adequate hemostasis.

procedures that are performed. Early ambulation is important to minimize the morbidity of surgery.

COMPLICATIONS

Intraoperative complications may include vascular and viscus injuries. The most common vascular injuries include injury to the epigastric artery, medial umbilical ligament, and accessory obturator vein but may also include the external iliac vessels and their tributaries. Viscus injuries include those to the ureters, bowel, and bladder. Take care to avoid injury to the obturator nerve. The incidence of all types of complications decreases with the increased experience of the operating surgeon and the surgeon's familiarity with the anatomy. Repair bladder and bowel injuries using intracorporeal techniques or open conversion, if necessary. Major injury to the iliac vessels should prompt vascular surgical consultation.

Postoperative complications may include hematomas, lymphocele, wound infection, ileus, small bowel obstruction, urinary retention, obturator nerve palsy, and deep venous thrombosis of the lower extremity.[8] To prevent deep venous thrombosis, administer prophylactic subcutaneous heparin or enoxaparin for 5 days beginning on postoperative day 1, and use sequential compression devices intraoperatively and postoperatively, if desired. Lymphocele is rare when a transperitoneal approach is used but is more common with an extraperitoneal approach. If a large lymphocele develops, perform drainage to avoid the increased risk of deep venous thrombosis.

SUMMARY

In conclusion, LPLND remains an important staging tool in the treatment of prostate cancer. With experience, this procedure can be performed with minimal morbidity and a low incidence of complications. Long-term studies will be necessary to define the potential curative effect of the node dissection for prostate cancer.

Tips and Tricks

- Sometimes the external iliac vein cannot be identified. Due to the compressive effects of the pneumoperitoneum the vein often appears flattened during laparoscopic surgery. The pneumoperitoneum can be temporarily decreased to 5 mm Hg to allow the vein to fill with blood in order to delineate the margins.

- If the internal inguinal ring cannot be identified, scrotal traction should move the spermatic cord and identify its entrance into the ring.
- On insertion of the laparoscopic port in the area of the inferior epigastric artery, significant bleeding may be encountered. Use the Carter-Thomasen CloseSure system to place a suture medial and lateral to the bleeding inferior epigastric vessel above and below the area of bleeding. These can be pulled tightly with a clamp during the surgery and then tied down onto the epigastric vessels after the completion of the procedure.
- If the Foley bag becomes distended like a balloon, suspect bladder injury due to dissection medial to the medial umbilical ligament. Identify bladder injury and repair with intracorporeal laparoscopic suturing techniques.
- There may be difficulty identifying medial boundary of nodal dissection. In this situation, firmly grasp the medial umbilical ligament with a grasping device and move it back and forth to delineate the obliterated umbilical artery. Use this as a starting point to begin blunt dissection to identify the medial edge of lymph node packet.

REFERENCES

1. Schuessler WW, Vancaillie TG, Reich H, Griffith DP: Transperitoneal endosurgical lymphadenectomy in patients with localized prostate cancer. J Urol 145:988–991, 1991.
2. Bhatta-Dhar, Reuther A, Zippe C, Klein E: No difference in six-year biochemical failure rates with or without pelvic lymph node dissection during radical prostatectomy in low-risk patients with localized prostate cancer. Urology 63:528–531, 2004.
3. Bader P, Burkhard F, Markwalder R, Studer U: Is a limited lymph node dissection an adequate staging procedure for prostate cancer? J Urol 168:514–518, 2002.
4. Daneshmand S, Quek M, Stein J, Skinner D: Prognosis of patients with lymph node–positive prostate cancer following radical prostatectomy: Long-term results. J Urol 172:2252–2255, 2004.
5. Kava B, Dalbagni G, Conlon K, Russo P: Results of laparoscopic pelvic lymphadenectomy in patients at high risk for nodal metastases from prostate cancer. Ann Surg Oncol 5:173–180, 1998.
6. Stone NS, Stock RG, Unger P: Laparoscopic pelvic lymph node dissection for prostate cancer: Comparison of the extended and modified techniques. J Urol 158:1891–1894, 1997.
7. Kerbl K, Clayman RV, Petros JA, et al: Staging pelvic lymphadenectomy for prostate cancer: A comparison of laparoscopic and open techniques. J Urol 150: 396–399, 1993.
8. Kavoussi L, Sosa E, Chandhoke P, et al: Complications of laparoscopic pelvic lymph node dissection. J Urol 149:322–325, 1993.

Laparoscopic Retroperitoneal Lymph Node Dissection

Mohamad E. Allaf

As many as 70% of men with clinical stage I nonseminomatous germ cell tumors (NSGCTs) undergo open retroperitoneal lymph node dissection (RPLND) or chemotherapy unnecessarily; thus, a minimally invasive approach to stage the retroperitoneum is attractive. Initial series of laparoscopic RPLND served this purpose and helped delineate those who have metastases and require chemotherapy versus those who can be observed safely. Because the probability of nodal disease posterior to the great vessels is minimal in the absence of anterior metastases, most series omitted the retrocaval and retroaortic dissections, and all patients found to have pathologic stage II disease received chemotherapy.[1]

Advances in instrumentation, the advent of hemostatic agents, and increased experience with laparoscopy within urology allowed the evolution of laparoscopic RPLND from a staging operation to a therapeutic one that fully duplicates the open technique. Retrocaval and retroaortic lymph nodes are now routinely excised in experienced centers, and chemotherapy is omitted for men harboring limited metastases.[2]

INDICATIONS AND CONTRAINDICATIONS

Approximately 30% of men with NSGCT with no radiographic evidence of lymph node metastases harbor occult nodal involvement at RPLND. Factors in the orchiectomy specimen predictive of occult lymph node involvement include lymphovascular involvement, percentage of embryonal component, and invasion of the rete testis or tunica albuginea.[3] The ideal candidate for laparoscopic RPLND has clinical stage I NSGCT (negative serum markers) and is at high risk of occult retroperitoneal disease. Patients at low risk for metastatic disease may also undergo laparoscopic RPLND, depending on their desires, especially if they are poor candidates for surveillance. A residual mass following chemotherapy in the setting of negative serum markers is another indication. These cases can be especially difficult due to the desmoplastic tissue reaction resulting from chemotherapy. Laparoscopic RPLND may also play a role in patients with gynecologic malignancy (cervical, endometrial, or ovarian) in specific circumstances.

Contraindications to laparoscopic RPLND are similar to those for the open approach. Patients with known bulky metastases and elevated tumor markers are typically not candidates for this approach. Prior abdominal surgery, previous peritonitis, and morbid obesity are not absolute contraindications, but these patients must be approached with great caution. Postchemotherapy laparoscopic RPLND (just like open RPLND), as mentioned previously, is technically challenging due to the obliteration of surgical planes and is associated with a higher probability of complications and open conversion.[4]

PATIENT PREOPERATIVE EVALUATION AND PREPARATION

All candidates for laparoscopic RPLND must have undergone a recent metastatic evaluation that, at minimum, includes a physical examination, serum tumor markers (lactate dehydrogenase, α-fetoprotein, and human chorionic gonadotropin), and a computed tomography (CT) scan of the chest, abdomen, and pelvis. Offer the patient the option to bank sperm preoperatively. Counsel all patients regarding the risks and benefits of the procedure and the possibility of open conversion. In the postchemotherapy setting, it is imperative to allow normalization of hematological parameters (white blood cells and platelets) and to optimize pulmonary function in patients who have received bleomycin.

Patients are given a mechanical bowel preparation the day before surgery to decompress the bowel. An enema may also be administered to cleanse the colon. Patients receive a first-generation cephalosporin such as cefazolin in the preoperative area. Thromboembolic deterrent stockings and sequential compression devices are placed on the lower extremities. An active type and screen must be available on all patients.

PATIENT POSITION AND OPERATING ROOM CONFIGURATION

After the induction of general anesthesia, place the patient in the supine position, pad the arms, and secure the arms to the patient's sides. Secure the patient's arms, chest, and hips to the table with wide cloth tape, allowing maximal rotation of the table during the procedure (Fig. 21–1). Perform a bilateral dissection, if needed, with this positioning scheme. Insert an orogastric tube and a Foley catheter before insufflation.

The surgeon and assistant stand on the side contralateral to the tumor, with the scrub nurse standing on the ipsilateral side. The surgeon is free to move to the other side during a bilateral dissection. Two monitors are used so that all members of the surgical team can observe the procedure (Fig. 21–2). A laparotomy set, including vascular clamps and retractors, is available for immediate access if needed.

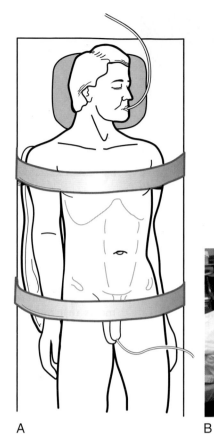

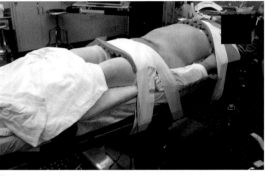

FIGURE 21–1. *A* and *B,* The patient is placed in the supine position with the arms adducted and pressure points padded. Wide cloth tape is used to secure the patient to the table.

A

B

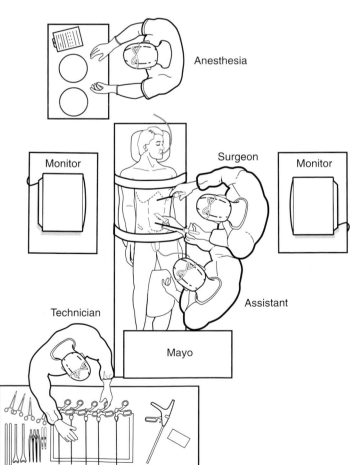

FIGURE 21–2. The surgeon stands on the side contralateral to the tumor. Two monitors are used so that all members of the team can observe the procedure. A laparotomy set is open and available for rapid access as needed to control severe bleeding.

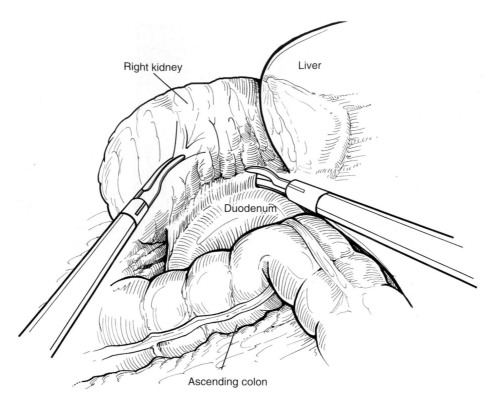

FIGURE 21–6. The duodenum is identified and a Kocher maneuver is performed with blunt and sharp dissection. The use of energy sources is minimized to avoid thermal damage to the duodenum. The inferior vena cava and renal hilum are exposed after the duodenum and colon are reflected medially.

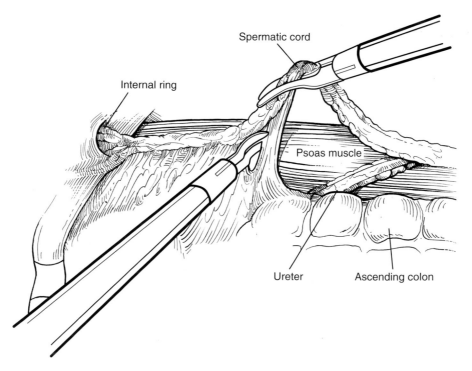

FIGURE 21–7. The ureter is identified as the gonadal vessels cross superiorly to reach the internal inguinal ring.

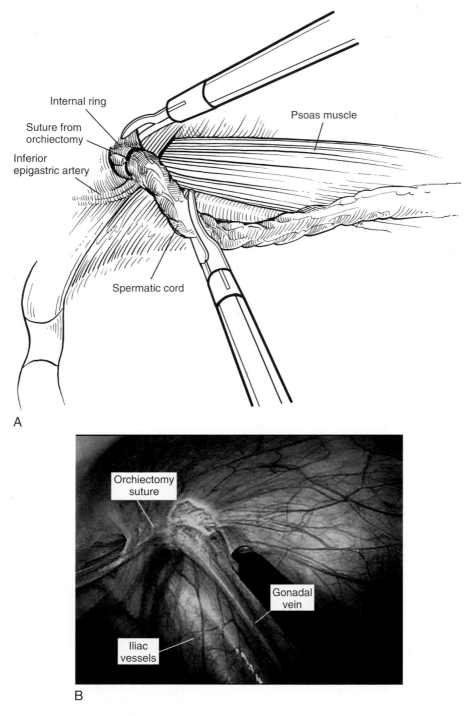

FIGURE 21–8. *A,* The orchiectomy suture is identified at the internal inguinal ring and electrocautery is used to incise the posterior peritoneum and circumferentially dissect the cord. *B,* The peritoneum is incised over the end of the spermatic cord at the internal inguinal ring.

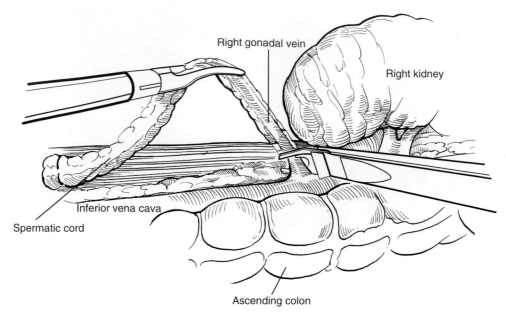

FIGURE 21–9. During a right-sided dissection, the cord is dissected to the origin of the gonadal vein at the vena cava. The vein is then clipped and divided at the level of the inferior vena cava.

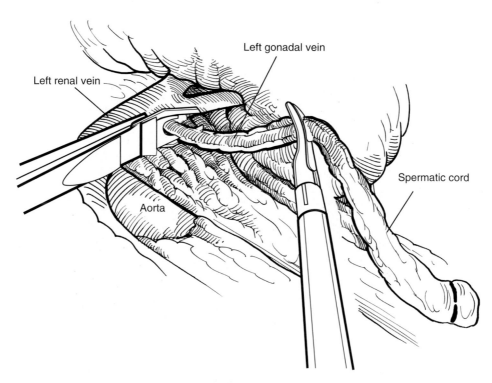

FIGURE 21–10. During a left-sided dissection, the cord is dissected to the origin of the gonadal vein at the left renal vein. The gonadal vein is then clipped and divided. The gonadal artery may be encountered and is also ligated and divided.

superiorly, ligate and divide it. If accessory lower pole renal vessels are encountered, do not injure them.

Precaval, Preaortic, and Lateral Dissection: "Split and Roll"

Gently lift the tissues overlying the great vessels and carefully score these tissues with electrocautery longitudinally (Fig.

21–11). Use blunt dissection to further aid in separating these lymphatic tissues along the length of the great vessels. This often creates a plane of dissection that can be developed laterally and helps in initiating the lateral dissection (Fig. 21–12). Although lumbar vessels can be encountered here, proceed laterally along the side wall and tackle these vessels later in the dissection. On the left side, only split the tissues to a level 5 cm inferior to the renal vein (origin of the inferior mesenteric

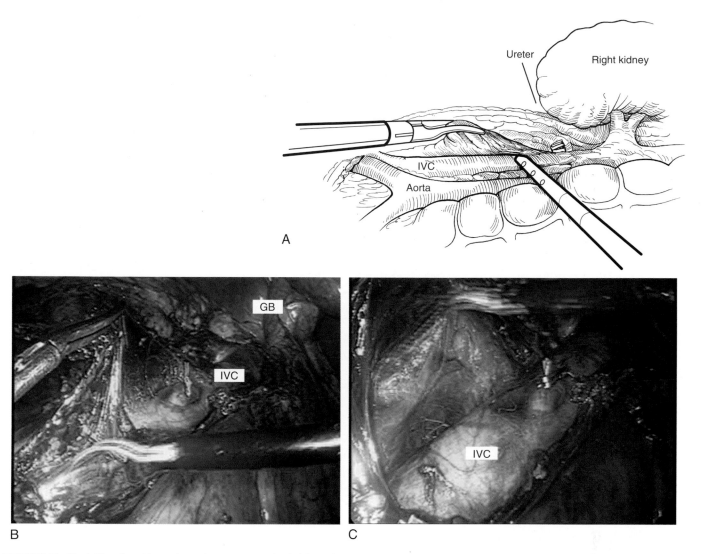

A

B

C

FIGURE 21–11. *A,* The adventitia overlying the vena cava is divided from the level of the renal vein to the bifurcation of the common iliac vessels. Electrocautery is used to longitudinally score the tissues and blunt dissection is used to further separate these tissues along the length of the inferior vena cava. *B,* The clips mark the site of transected gonadal vein. GB, gallbladder; IVC, inferior vena cava. *C,* The anterior surface of the vena cava is cleared of lymphatics and the gonadal vein clipped and divided on the surface of the vena cava. Using blunt and sharp dissection, the lymphatic tissue is then reflected laterally, toward the ureter.

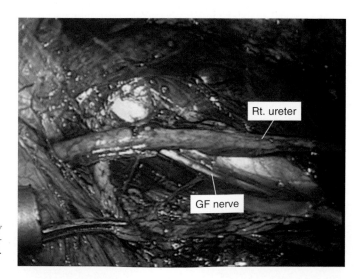

FIGURE 21–12. The dissection proceeds inferiorly, and the area bordered by the common iliac vessels and ureter is cleared of all lymphatic tissues. The genitofemoral (GF) nerve is seen in this view coursing anterior to the psoas muscle. Rt., right.

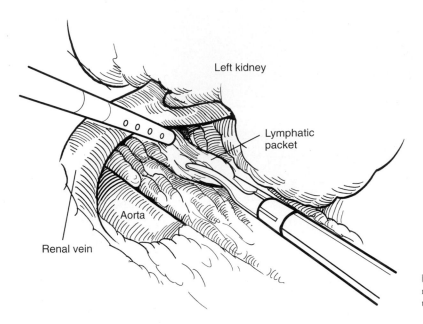

FIGURE 21–13. The renal artery and renal vein (including retroaortic veins) are always identified during the superior portion of this dissection and should not be confused for lumbar vessels.

artery) to avoid damage to the lumbar splanchnic nerves that may course into this region.

Lift the lateral nodal tissues and use the irrigation-suction device to gently separate these tissues from the underlying psoas fascia exposing small vessels and lymphatic channels. Ligate the lymphatic channels meticulously throughout the operation to minimize the risk of postoperative lymphocele formation. Carry the dissection superiorly to the renal vein, inferiorly to the common iliac vessels, and laterally to the ureter. Identify the sympathetic chains and leave them intact; do not mistake them for prominent lymphatic channels.

Interaortocaval Dissection

The paddle retractor is helpful in providing traction while medially rolling the remaining precaval/preaortic tissues to aid in their separation from the underlying great vessels. Identify the right renal artery and left renal vein (including retroaortic veins) during the superior portion of this dissection and do not confuse them for lumbar vessels (Fig. 21–13). Use blunt dissection with the irrigation-suction device to help define planes and separate nodal tissues from adjacent structures. Take particular care to avoid injury to the efferent sympathetic nerve fibers passing posterior to the IVC.

It is important to leave a long stump on the aorta/vena cava side when ligating lumbar vessels so that they can be grasped and controlled in the event a clip dislodges (Fig. 21–14). Lumbar vessels that retract into the iliopsoas muscle uncontrolled can usually be managed with pressure or a figure-of-eight stitch placed deep into the muscle. Lacerations of the IVC and aorta may occur during this operation and in the vast majority of cases do not mandate open conversion. Direct pressure usually prevents excessive hemorrhage and, in the case of venous bleeding, can achieve hemostasis without the need for additional maneuvers. Adjunct hemostatic agents also can be used successfully in this circumstance. If the bleeding persists or in the case of an aortotomy, direct pressure can be used temporarily before definitive repair is undertaken with intracorporeal suturing. In my experience, most venous lacerations

can be managed without the need for intracorporeal suture repair. It is important, however, not to manipulate the tissue after hemostasis is achieved via direct pressure. Return to this part of the dissection after a period of time, allowing the tear to adequately seal.

Retrocaval and Retroaortic Dissection

The posterior body wall lymphatic tissues remain at this point. Use closed atraumatic forceps or an irrigation-suction device to develop a plane between the posterior nodal tissues and great vessels (see Fig. 21–14). After ligation of posterior lumbar vessels, use the irrigation-suction device to retract the vena cava/aorta anteriorly. Finally, use an atraumatic grasper to lift the vena cava/aorta, and gently tease the nodal packet off the undersurface of the great vessel. Then laterally transpose the packet to conclude the dissection. Place the specimen in an EndoCatch bag and extract it. A drain is not routinely placed. At the conclusion of the procedure, the surgical template should be clear of all lymphatic tissues (Fig. 21–15). Inspect the abdomen carefully and remove all trocars under direct vision. Use a Carter-Thomason device to close all port sites to prevent hernia formation.

POSTOPERATIVE MANAGEMENT

The orogastric tube is removed in the operating room, and the urinary catheter is usually removed on the first postoperative day. Patients are routinely transferred to the floor following the procedure. Blood work including hemoglobin, white blood cell count, electrolytes, and creatinine is obtained on postoperative days 1 and 2. A liquid diet is started on the morning following surgery and advanced to a regular diet as tolerated. Patients ambulate on postoperative day 1 and are typically discharged on postoperative day 2. By 2 weeks following surgery, there should be no restrictions on activity level. Patients requiring chemotherapy can typically start adjuvant therapy soon after their operation.

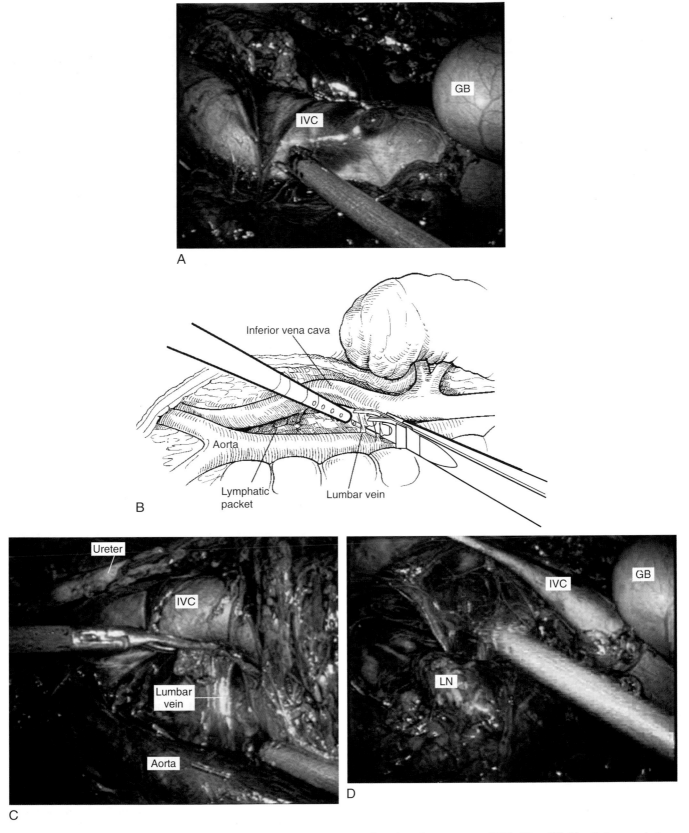

FIGURE 21–14. *A,* The precaval tissues are rolled medially to aid in their separation from the inferior vena cava (IVC). GB, gallbladder. *B,* Atraumatic forceps are used to develop a plane between the posterior nodal tissues and great vessels. Lumbar vessels interfering with the extraction of nodal tissues should be ligated and divided. It is important to leave a long stump on the aorta/vena cava side when clipping lumbar vessels so that they may be grasped and controlled in the event a clip dislodges. *C,* A grasper can be used to gently lift the vena cava/aorta so that the nodal packet can be teased off the undersurface of the great vessels. *D,* All retrocaval/retroaortic lymph nodes (LNs) are removed.

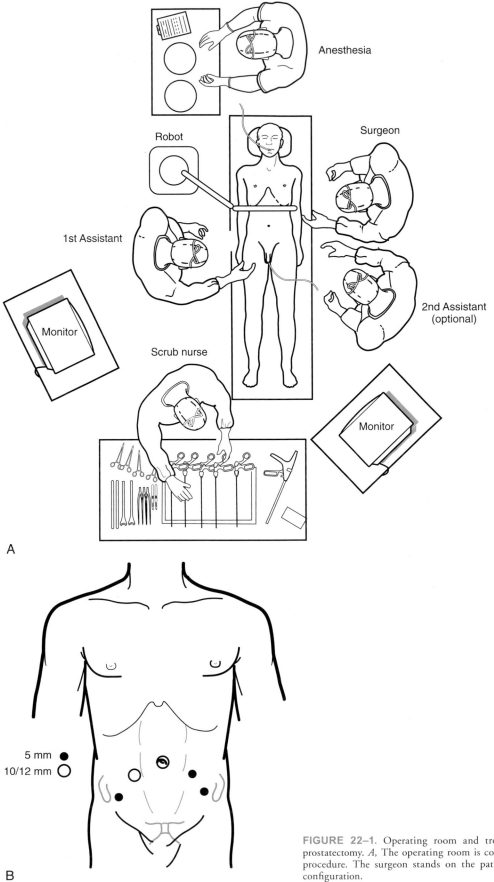

FIGURE 22–1. Operating room and trocar configuration for laparoscopic radical prostatectomy. *A,* The operating room is configured so that the entire team can see the procedure. The surgeon stands on the patient's left side. *B,* Our standard five-trocar configuration.

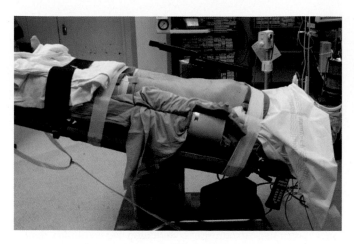

FIGURE 22–2. Patient positioning for transperitoneal laparoscopic radical prostatectomy. The patient's arms are tucked and padded at the sides with the operating table placed in the Trendelenburg position.

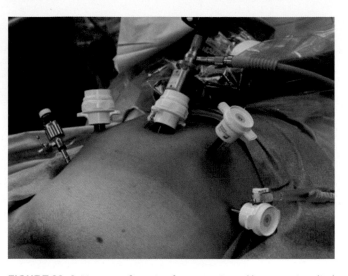

FIGURE 22–3. Trocor configuration for transperitoneal laparoscopic radical prostatectomy.

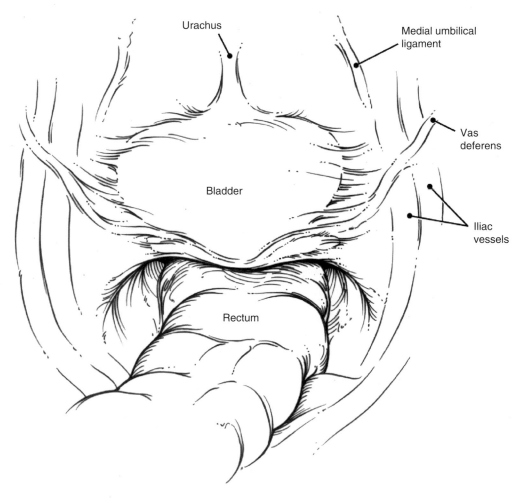

FIGURE 22–4. Initial intraperitoneal view detailing the relevant landmarks within the male pelvis during transperitoneal laparoscopic radical prostatectomy. (Drawn by Tim Phelps. Copyright © Johns Hopkins University.)

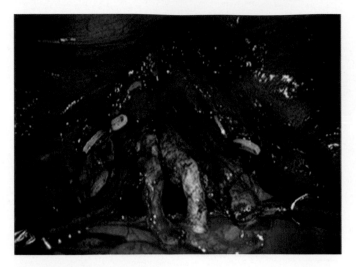

FIGURE 22–5. Seminal vesicle dissection. In lieu of using electrocautery for hemostasis, hemoclips are applied along the lateral aspect and tip of the seminal vesicle to secure the vascular pedicle and avoid thermal injury to the nearby neurovascular bundles. Completed bilateral seminal vesicle and vas dissection is shown.

Developing the Space of Retzius

Dissect the bladder from the anterior abdominal wall by dividing the urachus high above the bladder and incising the peritoneum bilaterally just medial to the medial umbilical ligaments using a hook electrocautery device. Applying cephalad and posterior traction on the urachus, identify and dissect the prevesical fat, exposing the space of Retzius (Fig. 22–7). Remove the fat overlying the anterior prostate, and coagulate the superficial branches of the dorsal venous complex (DVC) using bipolar electrocautery. Visible landmarks at this stage include the anterior aspect of the bladder and prostate, puboprostatic ligaments, endopelvic fascia, and pubic symphysis (Fig. 22–8). Sharply divide the endopelvic fascia and puboprostatic ligaments, exposing levator muscle fibers attached to the lateral and apical portions of the prostate. Meticulously and bluntly dissect these fibers from the surface of the prostate, exposing the prostatourethral junction.

Ligation of the Deep Dorsal Venous Complex

Ligate the deep DVC using a figure-of-eight 2-0 polyglactin GS21 suture, passing the needle beneath the DVC and anterior to the urethra (Fig. 22–9). Placing a 20-French metal van

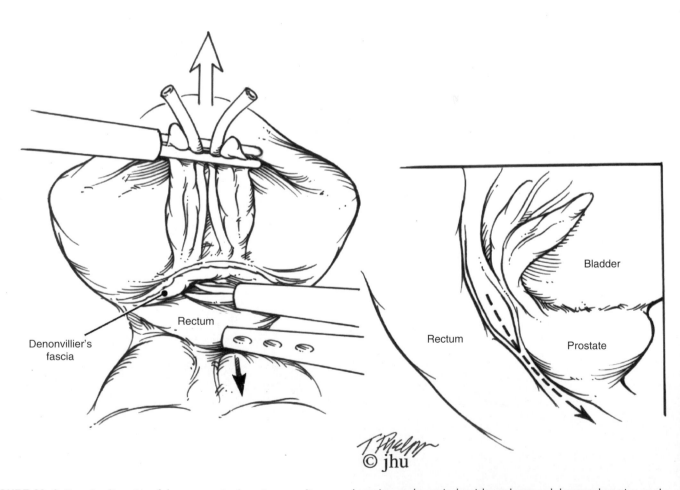

FIGURE 22–6. Posterior dissection of the prostate. As the assistant applies upward traction on the seminal vesicles and vasa and downward traction on the rectum, a transverse incision is made in Denonvillier's fascia below the seminal vesicles and blunt dissection is used to develop a plane between Denonvillier's fascia and the rectum. *Inset* demonstrates the direction of posterior dissection toward the prostatic apex. (Drawn by Tim Phelps. Copyright © Johns Hopkins University.)

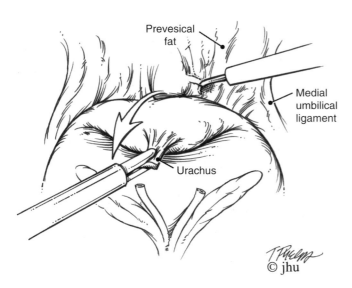

FIGURE 22–7. Division of urachus and entry into the space of Retzius. Cephalad and posterior traction on the urachus helps to identify the fatty alveolar tissue immediately anterior to the bladder, marking the proper plane of dissection. The medial umbilical ligaments demarcate lateral extent of the bladder dissection. (Drawn by Tim Phelps. Copyright © Johns Hopkins University.)

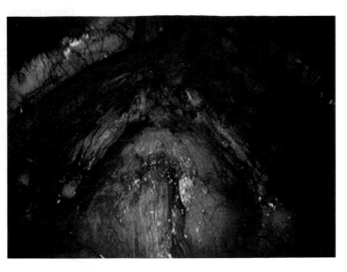

FIGURE 22–8. Retropubic view of the bladder and prostate following entry into the space of Retzius. The fatty tissue overlying the anterior aspect of the prostate has been removed, exposing the puboprostatic ligaments and endopelvic fascia.

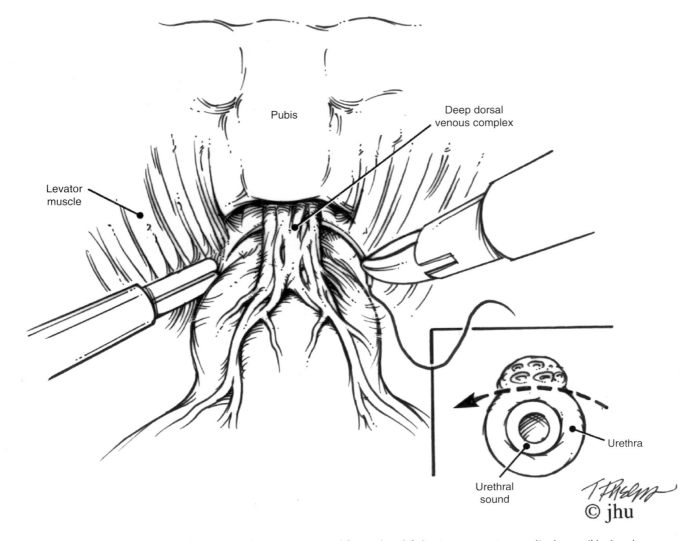

FIGURE 22–9. Ligation of the deep dorsal venous complex. A suture is passed from right to left, ligating the dorsal vein as distal as possible. *Inset* demonstrates the proper passage of the needle immediately anterior to the urethra. A urethral sound can be placed to ensure that the urethra is not incorporated in the suture. (Drawn by Tim Phelps. Copyright © Johns Hopkins University.)

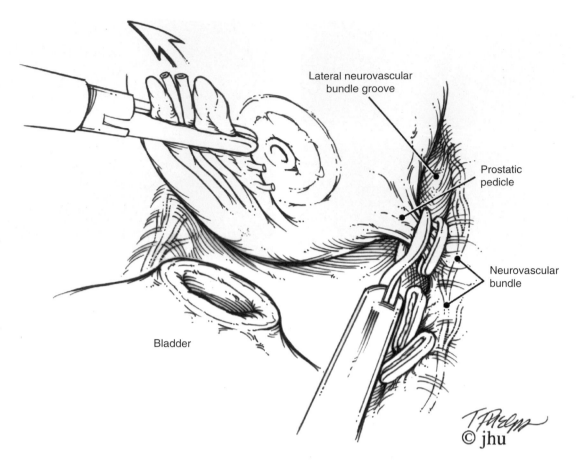

Lateral neurovascular
bundle groove

Prostatic
pedicle

Neurovascular
bundle

Bladder

FIGURE 22–14. Ligation of the right prostatic pedicle and antegrade dissection of the neurovascular bundle. With anterior traction on the seminal vesicles and vasa, the prostatic pedicles are identified and clipped and divided without electrocautery, staying close to the prostate surface. Direction and course of antegrade neurovascular bundle dissection are guided by the previously defined lateral neurovascular bundle groove. (Drawn by Tim Phelps. Copyright © Johns Hopkins University.)

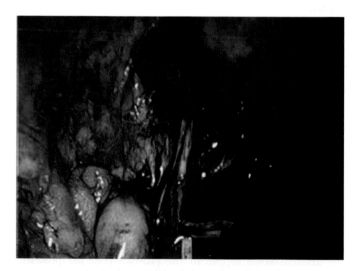

FIGURE 22–15. Antegrade dissection of the left neurovascular bundle. Intraoperative view demonstrating the fine V-shaped attachments between the left neurovascular bundle and the posterolateral surface of the prostate. Using both blunt and sharp dissection, the nerve bundle is gently swept off of the posterolateral surface of the prostate in the direction of the apex.

prostatic apex, resulting in an iatrogenic positive apical margin. Spot electrocautery may be required for minor bleeding from the DVC; avoid electrocautery immediately adjacent to the NVBs. Rarely, placement of additional DVC sutures is required if unexpected large venous sinuses are encountered. After complete division of the DVC, the anterior aspect of the prostato-urethral junction should be visible.

Prostatic Apical Dissection and Division of Urethra

The distal portion of the NVBs lie in intimate association with the lateral aspect of the prostatic apex; therefore, gently and meticulously dissect free the remaining attachments between the NVB and prostatic apex using a fine right-angled dissector and sharp dissection without electrocautery. By withdrawing the van Buren urethral sound into the prostatic urethra, the tip of the urethral sound can be useful for defining the precise junction between the prostatic apex and urethra, thus optimizing preservation of urethral length. Sharply divide the anterior urethra, taking care to avoid and preserve the NVBs coursing along the posterolateral surface of the urethra (Fig. 22–16). Before division of posterior urethra, take great care to inspect the contour of the posterior prostatic apex. In some patients,

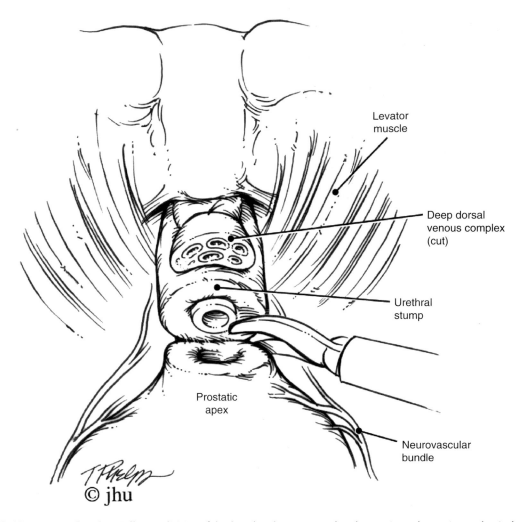

FIGURE 22–16. Division of urethra. Following division of the deep dorsal venous complex, the anterior and posterior urethra is sharply divided without electrocautery. Using the tip of a urethral sound, the precise point for transection of the urethra from the prostatic apex can be identified. (Drawn by Tim Phelps. Copyright © Johns Hopkins University.)

the anterior and posterior prostatic apex is asymmetric with protrusion of the posterior prostatic apex beneath the urethra. If not identified, transection of the posterior prostatic apex flush with the anterior margin may result in an iatrogenic posterior apical positive margin. Having already completed the posterior prostatic dissection, little additional dissection is typically required to free the prostate in its entirety once the posterior urethra and posterior striated urethral sphincter complex is divided.

Laparoscopic Inspection and Entrapment of the Prostate Specimen

Once the prostate is released completely, closely inspect the specimen margins laparoscopically. If there is concern about a positive margin, excise additional tissue and send it for frozen section at this time. If needed, temporarily place hemostatic gauze alongside the NVBs if small venous bleeding is identified and then remove the gauze before accomplishing the vesicourethral anastomosis. When indicated, perform laparoscopic bilateral pelvic lymph node dissection before accomplishing the anastomosis. Place the lymph node specimens

and the prostate in an entrapment sac and store them in the right lower quadrant of the abdomen until completion of the operation.

Vesicourethral Anastomosis

The critical first step in successfully accomplishing the vesicourethral anastomosis is to establish a secure posterior anastomosis, the site with the relatively greatest tension. Sutures along the posterior anastomosis are at risk for disruption with subsequent urinary leakage during passage of the urethral catheter if proper mucosa-to-mucosa approximation of the posterior anastomosis is not established. To avoid this complication, the assistant applies pressure to the perineum using a sponge stick to better reveal the posterior urethra. The assistant may also grasp the posterior bladder neck with a Maryland dissector or "hook" the trigone with the tip of a suction irrigator device in order to approximate the posterior bladder neck to the urethra. These maneuvers can reduce tension at the posterior anastomosis while the surgeon places and secures the sutures. Last, to further reduce tension at the anastomosis, release the lateral bladder attachments from the pelvic side

Incision of the Endopelvic Fascia and Dissection of Santorini's Plexus

Sweep the fatty tissue cephalad and lateral from the endopelvic fascia and from the anterior surface of the prostate. At this point, coagulate and divide the superficial dorsal vein. On both sides, laterally incise the endopelvic fascia toward the puboprostatic ligaments to its line of reflection. Peel the levator muscle attachments off the prostate, and perform the apical dissection to identify Santorini's plexus. Then divide the puboprostatic ligaments in contact with the pubic arch to facilitate dissection of Santorini's plexus. Start the apical dissection to identify the posterior limits of the plexus and the urethra.

Transection and Preservation of the Bladder Neck

Identify the bladder neck by palpating the supple bladder in comparison to the solid prostate. Pass a suture and secure it around the superficial tissue at the base of the prostate; leave a long tail for retraction. Insert a sixth trocar and place a toothed grasper on the stitch for upward traction of the bladder neck (Fig. 23–5). Incise the anterior aspect of the bladder neck at the limit between the muscular fibers of the detrusor and the prostatic capsule. When the bladder is opened, deflate the catheter balloon and pull the catheter tip out through the opening. Now place the grasper on the tip of the catheter. The assistant achieves countertraction by securing the catheter with a Kelly clamp placed just beyond the urethral meatus. In this manner, the assistant exposes the posterior edge of the prostate and the posterior bladder neck.

Transection of the bladder neck is completed. Place a locking grasper on the posterior bladder neck, which is retracted cephalad, exposing the anterior layer of Denonvillier's fascia (Fig. 23–6).

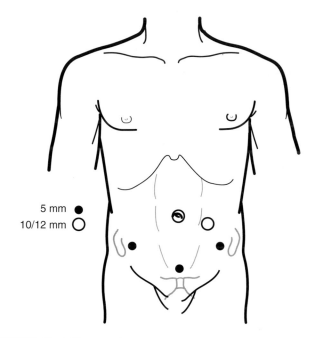

5 mm ●
10/12 mm ○

FIGURE 23–4. Trocar positioning.

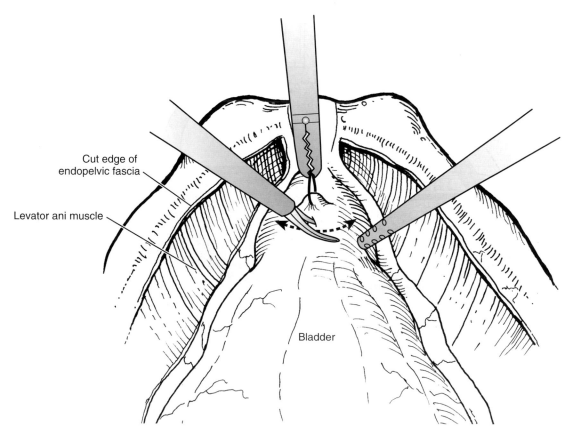

Cut edge of endopelvic fascia

Levator ani muscle

Bladder

FIGURE 23–5. Suspension of the base of the prostate and section of the anterior bladder neck.

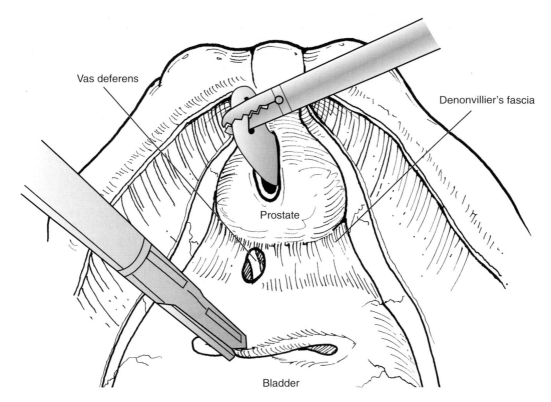

FIGURE 23–6. Division of the posterior bladder neck from the anterior layer of Denonvillier's fascia, which is incised transversely.

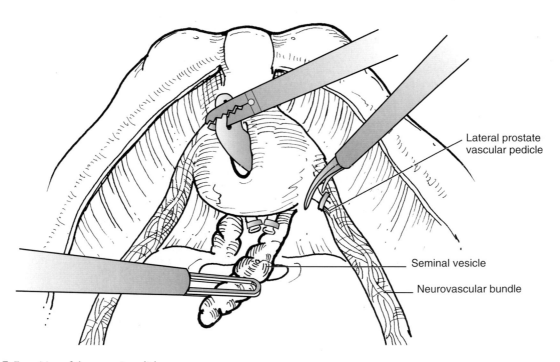

FIGURE 23–7. Exposition of the prostatic pedicles.

Dissection of Seminal Vesicles

Transversely incise the anterior layer of Denonvillier's fascia, which allows visualization of the vasa deferentia. Dissect, clip, and divide the vasa deferentia. Selectively clip and section the vascular pedicle for each structure. After division of each vas deferens, use upward traction on the distal portion of the vas to allow exposure of the seminal vesicles. Two large arteries are typically identified supplying each seminal vesicle from the lateral side (Fig. 23–7). Clip and divide these in a position immediately adjacent to the seminal vesicles. As each seminal vesicle is dissected, grasp these structures and pull them anteriorly. With anterior traction on the seminal vesicles, the prostatic pedicles are exposed.

Transection of Prostatic Pedicles and Preservation of Neurovascular Bundles

To optimize transection of prostatic pedicles and neurovascular bundle preservation, incise the visceral prostatic fascia and the lateral edge of the posterior Denonvillier's fascia in contact with prostatic capsule. Incision of the posterior layer of Denonvillier's fascia reveals prerectal fat and provides a safe plane of dissection (Fig. 23–8). Perform hemostasis of prostatic pedicles near the bundles with clips and near the prostatic capsule with bipolar electrocautery. After transection of the pedicles, open the plane between the neurovascular bundles and prostatic capsule. The last attachments of the bundles are small capsular arteries; divide them in a position immediately adjacent to the prostatic capsule after being controlled with clips. Extend dissection to the prostatic apex. Grasp the vasa deferentia and the seminal vesicles and retract them anteriorly. Medially complete incision of posterior Denonvillier's fascia, and dissect the prostatorectal plane behind the prostate to the rectourethral muscle.

Section of Santorini's Plexus and Section of Urethra

The assistant grasps the suture at the base of the prostate and retracts cephalad to put the apex on tension. Identify the margin between the urethra and dorsal vein complex, and place a figure-of-eight stitch around Santorini's plexus. Section the plexus perpendicularly. Then develop the plane between the plexus and the urethra in an oblique manner caudally. Incise the anterior urethral wall, and visualize the Foley catheter. Push the catheter through the anterior urethrotomy to open the urethral lumen and expose the posterior wall. The assistant retracts and rotates the prostate successively to each side and places the suction tip under the rectourethralis muscle and above the rectum. This maneuver allows a good exposure of the posterior lip of the prostatic apex, optimizing the section of posterior urethral wall and rectourethralis muscle and avoiding positive posterior margins. After incising the urethra and the rectourethralis muscle, place the freed prostate in an endoscopic bag. Extract the specimen through the slightly enlarged infra-umbilical port site after removing the Hasson cannula.

Vesicourethral Reconstruction

The Hasson cannula is now reinsected and the abdomen is insufflated. A posterior "tennis racket" reconstruction may be necessary in case of associated large prostatic hyperplasia or previous transurethral resection of the prostate. Perform the urethrovesical anastomosis using the method originally described by Van Velthoven.[11] Prepare the running suture by knotting together two 3-0 Vicryl 5/8 sutures of a total length of 14 cm (Fig. 23–9). Initiate the first running suture by placing a stitch outside-in through the bladder neck and inside-out on the urethra at the 4-o'clock position. Pass another needle outside-in through the bladder neck at the 3-o'clock position. Block the knot behind the bladder neck and place the needle on the right side of the operative field. Initiate the other running suture by placing a stitch symmetrical to the first at the 5-o'clock position. Leave the posterior lip of the bladder 2 cm apart from the urethral posterior wall. Complete the posterior anastomosis with four needle passages outside-in on the bladder and inside-out on the urethra, from the right to the left. When this is achieved, gently pull each suture on an alternating basis to approximate the bladder neck to the urethra. Then place a Foley catheter into the bladder. Peform the anterior anastomosis with the first suture outside-in on the bladder and inside-out on the urethra, from the right to the left. At the 10-o'clock position, knot the two running sutures on the outside of the bladder. Before inflating the balloon of the Foley catheter, make sure that it was not included in the running suture. Fill the bladder with 120 mL of saline in order to verify the integrity of the anastomosis.

Closure

Insert a small suction drain in the left lateral port site and place it in the Retzius space near the anastomosis. Close the anterior rectus fascia. Close skin incisions, and apply sterile dressings.

DISCUSSION

Initial development of the LRP was based on the experience of a few surgeons with transperitoneal laparoscopic access to the prostate and seminal vesicles.[3,6,12] Transperitoneal LRP was successfully introduced in routine clinical practice in France following the pioneering work of Gaston and Piéchaud in 1998 (unpublished series). This approach became predominant worldwide and is considered the "gold standard" of laparoscopic prostatectomy. However, other teams have shown that primary transperitoneal incision of the Douglas pouch is not indispensable for the dissection of the seminal vesicles. Through a transperitoneal access, Rassweiler and colleagues[5] proposed a technical alternative by approaching the Retzius space directly and by reproducing the retrograde technique described by Walsh. Using a purely preperitoneal approach, Raboy and associates[1] performed the seminal dissection after transection of the bladder neck.

Creation of a preperitoneal working space was initially described to perform laparoscopic inguinal hernia repair.[13] Since then, access to the preperitoneal space has been used for many other laparoscopic procedures, which include pelvic lymph node dissection, bladder neck suspension, varicocelectomy, and, more recently, radical prostatectomy.[1,13] Presently, creation of a preperitoneal space is standardized and represents a minimally invasive approach to the prostate. We developed a technique with initial blunt finger dissection, which is a fast, safe, and less costly alternative to the balloon technique.[13] Performing this dissection anterior to the posterior rectus sheath minimizes the risk of inadvertent entry into the peritoneal cavity.

All crucial elements of our previously described transperitoneal technique of LRP[14] are reproduced, and only a few technical points have been modified since we switched to the extraperitoneal approach. Trocar geometry is similar to that previously described in transperitoneal LRP, but a sixth trocar can be introduced during initial space creation. This 5-mm suprapubic trocar does not result in any additional morbidity, but we have found it useful when mobilizing the prostate (see Fig. 23–4). Dissection of the prostate is performed in a traditional anterograde fashion and allows preservation of the neurovascular bundles. During this step, we prefer to use clips rather than any kind of thermal energy to achieve hemostasis.

Based on our favorable experience with two hemicircumferential running sutures when performing the vesicourethral

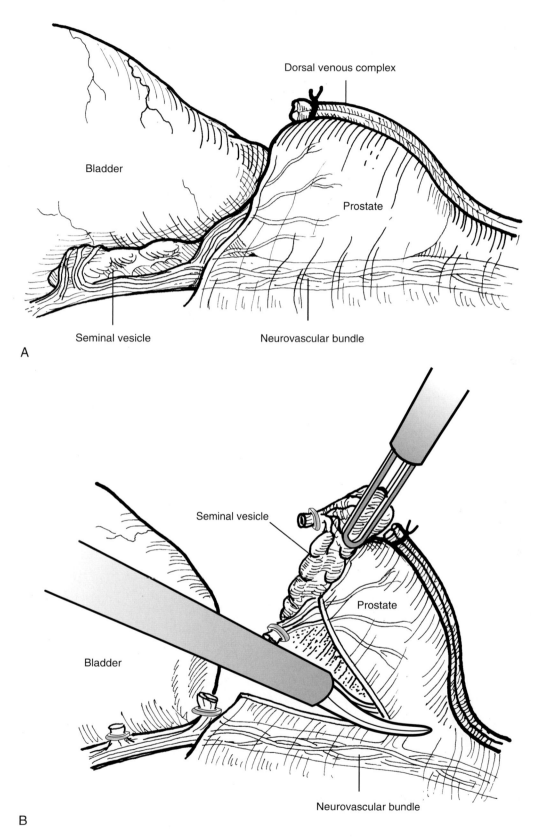

FIGURE 23–8. *A–C,* Section of prostatic pedicles and preservation of neurovascular bundles.

Continued

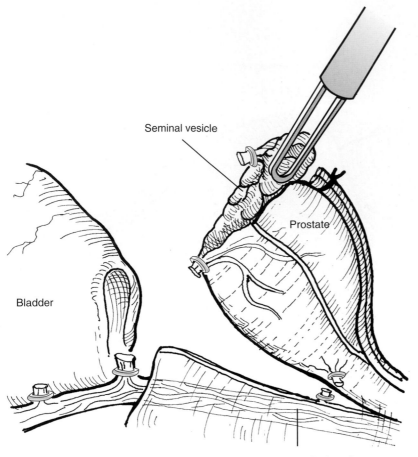

C

FIGURE 23–8, cont'd.

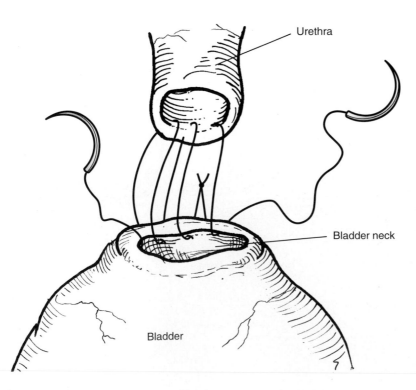

FIGURE 23–9. Vesicourethral reconstruction: needle passages of the posterior anastomosis.

reconstruction,[15] we recently adopted a modification proposed by Van Velthoven and colleagues.[11] The latter technique requires only one intracorporeal knot instead of three and simplifies the control of the posterior half of the anastomosis because all the posterior stitches are placed before approximating the bladder neck to the urethra.

Many teams have now reported that opening of the peritoneal cavity is not indispensable.[8–10,16] In addition, several arguments support the use of a purely extraperitoneal approach. Risks of intraperitoneal injuries during access creation are minimized. Bowel adherences due to previous abdominal surgery do not necessitate any particular modification or precaution when creating the preperitoneal access. Previous inguinal herniorraphy with mesh, while not a contraindication to extraperitoneal LRP, does increase the complexity of prevesical space development, and in these cases, pelvic lymphadenectomy is often impossible.

Other potential advantages of avoiding peritoneal entry are to limit the risk of postoperative ileus and to limit postoperative pain. In comparing extraperitoneal LRP to transperitoneal LRP at our center, measures of perioperative morbidity (postoperative pain, time to full diet) were more favorable when using the extraperitoneal technique.[10] In transperitoneal LRP, some urine and blood inevitably enter the peritoneal cavity during the intervention, causing at least some degree of chemical peritonitis. During the postoperative period, urinary extravasation through the anastomosis is not exceptional and occasionally can become a morbid complication. In 10% to 17.2% of patients, persistent urine in the suction drain can be present for more than 6 days due to anastomotic leakage.[17–19] To what extent such a urinary leak can communicate with the peritoneal cavity is unclear; however, this mechanism can lead to more severe complications. In transperitoneal laparoscopic series, prolonged ileus attributed to anastomotic leak was reported in 2.8% to 8.6% of cases.[7,19] In a large series, secondary anastomotic leakage was diagnosed after catheter removal in a context of acute pain, acute urinary retention, and peritoneal irritation syndrome in 2% of patients.[17] Ileus, anastomotic leak, and hemoperitoneum are all classified in the second group of the complication grading system proposed by Clavien and colleagues for laparoscopic surgery.[17,20] Grade II complications are "potentially life threatening but without residual disability."

Establishing the complexity and technical difficulty of a surgical intervention is mostly a subjective exercise. However, indirect data suggest that the extraperitoneal approach may provide a simplification of laparoscopic prostatectomy. Presently, there are only a few comparative studies dealing with transperitoneal versus extraperitoneal LRP.[10,21] Uniformly, all these studies have shown a statistically significant decrease in operative time ranging from 10 to 54 minutes, which suggests that extraperitoneal LRP may be a more straightforward procedure.

Furthermore, especially in the learning curve phase, open conversion to radical prostatectomy can be performed in the familiar environment of the retropubic space. But even without the necessity of conversion, for those who begin performing laparoscopic prostatectomy, complications (leak or hemorrhage) will be also easier to manage when using the extraperitoneal approach.

The first results of extraperitoneal LRP in terms of oncologic cure and preservation of continence and potency do not seem to differ from those of transperitoneal LRP.[10,16,22] This technique seems reproducible, with possibly a decrease in operative time.[10,21,23] These advantages are essential in a university center like ours, especially because teaching LRP is a complex process requiring a large number of cases (>50) to reach the plateau of a learning curve.[24] Using an extraperitoneal approach, the first two steps do not require a long experience, and the rest of the procedure uses familiar anatomic landmarks, which are the same as for retropubic access. Furthermore, compared with the transperitoneal approach, this technique needs only one space of dissection instead of two. In our experience, teaching LRP with this technique has also become easier. Also, we believe that the extraperitoneal approach may improve the learning curve of LRP, which is essential to its development.

Despite all these arguments, unanswered questions remain. Obviously, the primary goal of radical prostatectomy is oncologic cure and preservation of urinary continence and potency. Attempts to decrease operative time and perioperative morbidity should not outrival these principles. The task that remains is to prospectively compare the two techniques considering all these outcome variables in order to objectively determine the relative merits of each of these approaches.

SUMMARY

LRP is undergoing a continuous technical development. At our center, the extraperitoneal approach appears to be the logical evolution for LRP because it combines the advantages of laparoscopic surgery and retropubic access and significantly reduces operative time. This technique is well standardized, but further evaluation of long-term results is necessary. We believe the extraperitoneal technique may shorten the learning curve of LRP.

REFERENCES

1. Raboy A, Albert P, Ferzli G: Early experience with extraperitoneal endoscopic radical retropubic prostatectomy. Surg Endosc 12:1264, 1998.
2. Schuessler WW, Schulam PG, Clayman RV, et al: Laparoscopic radical prostatectomy: Initial short-term experience. Urology 50:854, 1997.
3. Guillonneau B, Vallancien G: Laparoscopic radical prostatectomy: The Montsouris technique. J Urol 163:1643, 2000.
4. Abbou CC, Salomon L, Hoznek A, et al: Laparoscopic radical prostatectomy: Preliminary results. Urology 55:630, 2000.
5. Rassweiler J, Sentker L, Seemann O, et al: Heilbronn laparoscopic radical prostatectomy. Technique and results after 100 cases. Eur Urol 40:54, 2001.
6. Kavoussi LR, Schuessler WW, Vancaillie TG, et al: Laparoscopic approach to the seminal vesicles. J Urol 150:417, 1993.
7. Dahl DM, L'esperance JO, Trainer AF, et al: Laparoscopic radical prostatectomy: Initial 70 cases at a U.S. university medical center. Urology 60:859, 2002.
8. Dubernard P, Benchetrit S, Chaffange P, et al: Prostatectomie extra-péritonéale rétrograde laparoscopique (P.E.R.L) avec dissection première des bandelettes vasculo-nerveuses érectiles. Technique simplifiée—à propos de 100 cas. Prog Urol 13:163, 2003.
9. Stolzenburg JU, Do M, Pfeiffer H, et al: The endoscopic extraperitoneal radical prostatectomy (EERPE): Technique and initial experience. World J Urol 20:48, 2002.
10. Hoznek A, Antiphon P, Borkowski T, et al: Assessment of surgical technique and perioperative morbidity associated with extraperitoneal versus transperitoneal laparoscopic radical prostatectomy. Urology 61:617, 2003.
11. Van Velthoven RF, Ahlering TE, Peltier A, et al: Technique for laparoscopic running urethrovesical anastomosis: The single knot method. Urology 61:699, 2003.

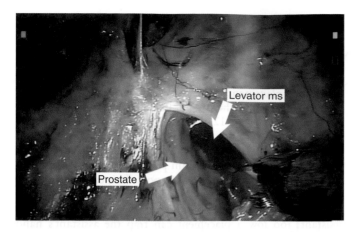

FIGURE 24–4. Clear definition of levator side wall from prostate is key to a bloodless dissection. The lowest point of the incision should expose a small amount of perivesical fat. This is a signal that the incision has been taken sufficiently proximal. ms, muscle.

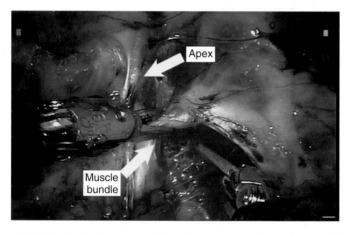

FIGURE 24–5. This very consistent bundle is usually cauterized with bipolar energy before division from the prostate to help minimizing bleeding.

Entering the Endopelvic Fascia

Sharply incise the fascia laterally so that the underlying prostate capsule and levator muscles are seen (Fig. 24–4). Initiate this incision in the region of the prostatovesical junction and then carry it toward the apex of the prostate. This helps avoid bleeding from the vessels that are consistently present more apically.

Inferior and lateral to the apex of the prostate, a band of muscle is consistently present that usually encases a vein or artery or both. Remove this band from the prostate by first applying bipolar energy to the bundle very near its insertion to the prostate and then dividing it with scissors (Fig. 24–5). With the prostate apex clearly in view, thin the fascia overlying the dorsal venous complex (DVC) in order to define the junction between the vein and the urethra. Once this is achieved, divide the DVC.

Ligation of the Dorsal Venous Complex

The DVC can be handled by one of several methods; the most common is either suture ligation or stapling. If suturing is to be performed, a 0-Vicryl on a CT-1 needle is typically used to place a figure-of-eight around the DVC. Often, a back-bleeding suture is also placed toward the prostate. Once tied, the DVC can be divided at this point, but many surgeons leave this intact temporarily until the urethra is approached later during the case. I prefer to staple the DVC using the Ethicon laparoscopic stapler with a 45-mm cartridge length and 2.5-mm staple leg length. (Ethicon Endo-Surgery). Introduce the stapler into the field through the lateral 12-mm port. From this angle, place the anvil portion of the stapler on the contralateral side so that the black lines just pass the edge of the DVC (Fig. 24–6). Use of a 22-French Foley helps prevent stapling of the urethra because this diameter catheter is very difficult to fit inside the open jaws of the stapler. Clamp the stapler to the locked position and hold it for 10 seconds before firing. This provides tissue compression, which improves staple formation and hemostasis. Once divided, there should be a small line of stapled tissue left, which can be easily divided later. If there is any bleeding or if the staple line separates, use a small figure-of-eight stitch with a 3-0 Vicryl to stop the remaining bleeding.

Prostatovesical Junction

Switch the lens to a 30-degree down lens to provide a more familiar downward view of the prostatovesical junction. The tableside assistant then slowly pushes in and withdraws the Foley catheter. The prior removal of superficial fat usually allows easily visualization of the catheter balloon. Once the location of the junction is firmly in mind, perform sharp dissection with either cautery or scissors just cranial to the junction (Fig. 24–7). Carry the dissection from medial to lateral; if it is done carefully, the large superficial veins coursing from the prostate to the bladder can be lifted off the underlying structures, minimizing bleeding. The lateral junction between the prostate and the bladder is then visualized.

From this point, carry the dissection from lateral to medial to thin out the attachment fibers. Enter the bladder neck, and withdraw the balloon of the Foley catheter. Grasp the catheter through its eye with the fourth arm and pull the catheter anteriorly. Leave the posterior lip of the bladder neck intact while dividing the remaining lateral fibers that are attaching the bladder to the prostate. In many cases, this dissection can be carried posterior to the bladder neck, thereby preserving the circular fibers of the bladder neck, which may aid in early continence recovery.

Finally, completely divide the bladder neck. Inspect the bladder neck to ensure that there is sufficient distance from the ureteral orifices for later suturing and to identify any need for later bladder neck reconstruction. Indigo carmine is not routinely administered during this dissection.

Seminal Vesicles and Vas Ligation

After the bladder neck is divided at the proper level, note a whitish fibrous layer. Divide this layer; in some patients, it is quite thick. Immediately posterior to this layer is a layer of fat overlying the ampulla of the vas. It is helpful at this point of the dissection to observe the general size of the prostate (Fig.

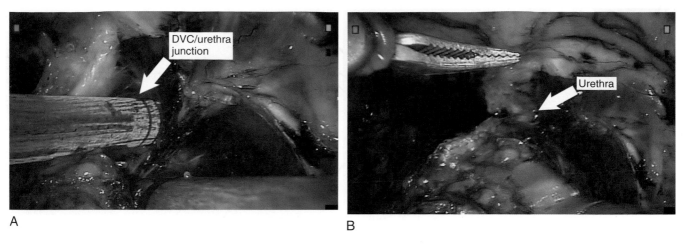

FIGURE 24–6. *A* and *B,* The second black line is placed at the junction between the dorsal venous complex (DVC) and urethra. If this is not performed the residual staple line is more likely to split slightly and bleed.

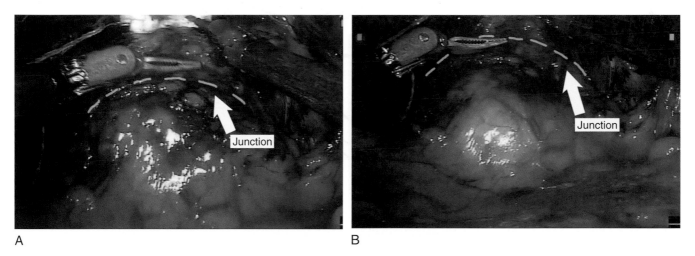

FIGURE 24–7. *A* and *B,* Movement of the Foley balloon (inflated to 10 mL) in and out greatly aids in the identification the prostatovesical junction. If an eccentric movement of the catheter balloon is observed, a large median lobe is likely present.

24–8). If the prostate is very large or has a significant median lobe component, then the angle at which this layer is divided is much steeper than if the prostate is small. If this is not appreciated, for example, in the case of large prostate, a portion of the prostate may easily be shaved off as one is searching for the vasa if too shallow a plane is taken.

Once the ampullae are identified and dissected, excise long sections. Do this by dissecting sufficient tissue away from the lateral sides of the vasa and then grasping one firmly with the fourth robotic arm. Use upward traction to bring more of the vas into better view, then further dissect it (Fig. 24–9). Use the long excised remnants as a pledget during the anastomosis. Once the vasa are divided, pull the stumps on the prostate upward using the fourth arm to visualize the medial aspects of the seminal vesicles. The bulk of the vasculature to the seminal vesicles courses laterally; thus, medial dissection is easier and allows the seminal vesicles to be rolled upward and medially. Often, very little dissection then needs to be performed laterally. My preference is to use a bipolar grasper and scissors during this dissection to allow precise division of the vessels, minimizing any possible damage to the nearby neurovascular bundles.

Prostate Dissection

Grasp the stumps of the vasa with the fourth arm and use them to pull the prostate upward toward the pubis and out of the pelvis toward the umbilicus. Once proper traction is obtained, note the posterior contour of the prostate (Fig. 24–10). Incising Denonvillier's fascia precisely at this point helps to minimize any chance of injuring the rectum or incising into the prostate. Divide the fascia along the posterior surface of the prostate, and gently push down the fat overlying the rectum, away from the prostate. Definitely identify the posterior capsule of the prostate, and carry this plane of dissection toward the urethra as far as can be reached. In men with smaller prostates, often the fibers of the rectourethralis can be identified. Once the rectum has been definitely mobilized, either resect or spare the cavernous nerves. For a non–nerve-sparing procedure, the plane adjacent to the rectum can be continued laterally. This provides a large margin around the base and lateral portion of the prostate (Fig. 24–11).

For a nerve-sparing procedure, closely follow the capsule of the prostate from medial to lateral. First, either the fourth arm

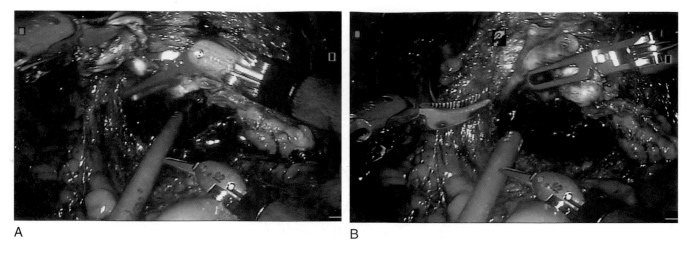

FIGURE 24–12. *A,* The seminal vesicles are useful handles for retraction. *B,* Grasping these structures at their insertion into the prostate helps to prevent inadvertent tearing.

plane opens up very easily and the remaining bundle can be teased away with very little difficulty.

Several different methods have been described to control bleeding around the pedicle, including bipolar cautery and sharp dissection, hemostatic clips, and even placement of bulldog clamps on the pedicles with later oversewing.[5] Intuitively, minimizing energy discharge in the region of the pedicles seems the most prudent; this idea has been supported by experimental work in the canine model.[6] However, clinical outcomes are awaited to support the optimal method for sparing the neurovascular bundle. As the dissection is continued to the apex of the prostate, one must be aware of the proximity of the rectum to the apex of the prostate. Therefore, it is again of great importance to maximize the posterior dissection of the prostate to the apex *before* the lateral dissection is performed, if possible. Once the apex is reached, the anterior urethra is dissected from surrounding tissue. If staples were used to ligate the DVC, a short burst of monopolar cautery expeditiously divides the tissue, allowing the underlying urethra to come into view. The monopolar device is immediately switched out, and cold scissors are used to further dissect the notch of the prostate. The urethra is entered with scissors, and the Foley catheter is withdrawn until it is just visible in the stump of the urethra. The fourth arm is then used to gradually rock the prostate back and forth to provide exposure for division of the posterior urethra and remaining rectourethral attachments. Once freed, the prostate is then entrapped in an entrapment sac and placed in the upper abdomen until the anastomosis is complete.

Urethrovesical Anastomosis

For the anastomosis, I prefer to use the Van Velthoven stitch.[7] This running, double-armed suture has many benefits, including minimizing knot-tying and providing a water-tight anastomosis. The suture consists of 3-0 monocryl sutures tied at the loose ends with a length of 6 to 7 inches for each arm. The needles can be a UR-6, RB-1 but I prefer an SH needle. Once the holding knot is tied, a very small piece of vas is placed as a pledget to bolster the posterior bladder neck. Alternatively,

Lapra-Ty can be used (Ethicon Endo-Surgery, Cincinnati, OH).

Start the suture by placing both arms of the suture outside-in at the 6-o'clock position. As a routine, I change the camera back to the 0-degree lens at this point to provide a better view of the urethra. Place the sutures on the urethra inside-out at the 6-o'clock position. Use the right arm of the suture to go outside-in on the bladder, inside on the urethra, outside on the bladder so that the suture exits at about 3 o'clock on the bladder neck. Then slowly but firmly pull the sutures upward so that the bladder neck can be brought into close apposition to the urethra. At this point the vas bolster helps to prevent the knot from "sawing" across the posterior bladder neck. Use the fourth arm to hold the 3-o'clock suture taut, thus anchoring the bladder neck to the urethra. Suture the left-hand suture in the same manner until it exits inside-out on the urethra at the 11-o'clock position. Then lock this suture in the fourth arm and sew the right hand suture to the 1-o'clock position inside-out on the urethra. Pass the transition suture at 12 o'clock outside-in on the urethra and pass it inside-out on the bladder neck. Pass the catheter into the bladder. Tie the suture across the anastomosis. Irrigate with 120 mL of saline via the Foley catheter to test for watertightness. If there is no leak or a small leak, do not place a drain. If a drain is left, it could easily be left through the lateral robot port site.

Exiting

Place the specimen retrieval bag string totally into the abdomen under direct vision. Then remove the camera from the port and place the bag into the lateral 12-mm port site. Place a laparoscopic needle driver into the camera port site, and remove the bag drawstring from the abdomen. Clamp the string with a hemostat. Undock the robot. Remove the trocars under direct vision to check for any bleeding. Remove the specimen by extending the incision of the camera port site to about 4 cm. Open the fascia with cautery until the specimen can be retrieved. Close the port sites with a subcuticular stitch of 3-0 or 4-0 Vicryl, and close the skin with a skin adhesive (Dermabond, Ethicon, Somerville, NJ) or stitches and Steristrips.

POSTOPERATIVE MANAGEMENT

Remove the orogastric tube in the operating suite. Patients are prescribed ketorolac and morphine as needed for pain. Patients are encouraged to ambulate as soon as possible, usually within 6 hours of returning to their hospital room. A clear liquid diet is instituted that is advanced to a regular diet by the patient's next meal. Discharge is planned for the morning of postoperative day 1. Patients are seen back in 1 week for catheter removal.

COMPLICATIONS

All complications related to laparoscopic surgery readily apply to robotic prostatectomy. Intraoperative complications include bleeding, injury to adjacent organs, and conversion to open surgery. Rectal injury is an ever-present danger, especially in patients with a history of preoperative androgen ablation. In cases of small rectal tears, consideration can be given to primary closure in two layers with interrupted permanent sutures in patients who have been given a preoperative bowel preparation. Copious irrigation of the pelvis and broad-spectrum intravenous antibiotics should be instituted. Large injuries may be handled by conversion to an open procedure with primary rectal repair and consideration of a diverting ileostomy. Postoperative hematuria may be troublesome for some patients. Instruct patients to seek immediate attention for problems involving catheter obstruction related to clot retention. Late complications such as incontinence and impotence are beyond the scope of this chapter but are explained in detail in other sources.

Tips and Tricks

- Meticulous port site selection is the key for allowing adequate working space between the robotic arms. This enables maximum range of motion of the arms, thereby maximizing mobility.
- Clean away the superficial fat over the surface of the prostatovesical junction as completely as possible to enable visualization of the junction.
- The fourth arm provides excellent steady retraction of the vasa, seminal vesicles, and prostate, thereby enabling rapid anterior dissection of the seminal vesicles and precise dissection of the neurovascular bundles. Make every effort to maximize use of the fourth arm.
- Small, frequent camera movements are essential for precise dissection and decreasing operating room times.

REFERENCES

1. Abbou CC, Hoznek A, Salomon L, et al: Laparoscopic radical prostatectomy with a remote controlled robot. J Urol 165:1964–1966, 2001.
2. Menon M, Shrivastava A, Tewari A, et al: Laparoscopic and robot assisted radical prostatectomy: Establishment of a structured program and preliminary analysis of outcomes. J Urol 168:945–949, 2002.
3. Sarle R, Tewari A, Shrivastava A, et al: Surgical robotics and laparoscopic training drills. J Endourol 18:63–66; discussion 66–67, 2004.
4. Pick DL, Lee DI, Skarecky DW, et al: Anatomic guide for port placement for da Vinci robotic radical prostatectomy. J Endourol 18:572–575, 2004.
5. Ahlering TE, Eichel L, Chou D, et al: Feasibility study for robotic radical prostatectomy cautery-free neurovascular bundle preservation. Urology 65:994–997, 2005.
6. Ong AM, Su LM, Varkarakis I, et al: Nerve-sparing radical prostatectomy: Effects of hemostatic energy sources on the recovery of cavernous nerve function in a canine model. J Urol 172:1318–1322, 2004.
7. Van Velthoven RF, Ahlering TE, Peltier A, et al: Technique for laparoscopic running urethrovesical anastomosis: The single knot method. Urology 61:699–702, 2003.

CHAPTER 25

Laparoscopic Radical Cystectomy and Urinary Diversion

Andrew A. Wagner
Christian P. Pavlovich

Radical cystectomy with urinary diversion remains the preferred treatment for localized, invasive bladder carcinoma.[1] Beginning in the early 1990s, several urologists investigated the use of laparoscopy as an access technique to perform both extirpative and reconstructive procedures, including radical cystectomy. With improvements in instrumentation and laparoscopic training, more urologists are performing laparoscopic radical cystectomy (LRC); however, it remains an extremely challenging procedure even when performed by experienced laparoscopic surgeons.

Laparoscopic cystectomy was first performed in 1992 by Parra and colleagues for a 27-year-old paraplegic with pyocystis.[2] The first reported LRC for cancer was performed in 1993.[3] Since then there have been numerous descriptions of LRC technique, most of which describe relatively minor variations in the extirpative component of the case.[4–9] The majority of reported cases have involved male patients, although LRC has been performed on female patients. Moinzadeh and colleagues[10] reported their experience in 11 female patients and described the use of a vaginal and uterine manipulator to facilitate the procedure. They were able to successfully perform both anterior exenteration (7 patients) and female organ–sparing cystectomy (4 patients).

The urinary diversion is performed following the cystectomy and can be fashioned either through an open incision, purely laparoscopically, or through a combination of both techniques. As for open surgery, many variations of urinary diversion have been described, including cutaneous ureterostomies, ileal conduit, continent cutaneous reservoir, orthotopic neobladder, and rectosigmoid pouch with ureterosigmoidostomies.

The original reports of laparoscopic-assisted ileal conduits described the extracorporeal creation of the ureteroileal anastomosis through either a small flank or midline incision.[11] More recently, complete intracorporeal creation of the ileal reanastomosis and ureteroileal anastomoses has been described. Gill and colleagues[12] reported the first completely intracorporeal radical cystectomy and urinary diversion by ileal conduit. Two men underwent the procedure for muscle invasive bladder cancer. Operating times were 11.5 and 10 hours, and there were no complications.

Laparoscopic or open rectosigmoid pouch has also been performed after LRC.[5,9] This allows the patient a continent reservoir and avoids an ileal resection and anastomosis but confers with it the concern for later malignancy at the ureterosigmoid junctions, as well as the problems associated with frequent watery stools.

For many urologists, orthotopic ileal neobladder has become the preferred method of diversion in appropriate candidates. Laparoscopic urologists have therefore had a natural progression toward attempting to incorporate this method of diversion into their armamentarium. Most groups to date have completed the neobladder through a midline or Pfannenstiel incision following laparoscopic cystectomy.[4,6] Basillote and associates[4] compared LRC with an ileal neobladder created through a 15-cm Pfannenstiel incision to patients undergoing traditional open radical cystectomy with neobladder creation. They found there was less postoperative pain and a shorter hospitalization in the LRC patients. Others have performed part[13] or all[7] of the neobladder intracorporeally. Gill and colleagues[14] investigated a completely intracorporeal ileal neobladder in a porcine model. They fashioned a neobladder with a Studer limb in 12 animals with generally good success. The same group has reported on their human experience with complete intracorporeal orthotopic ileal neobladder in two patients. The operative time was 8.5 and 10.5 hours. Both patients had daytime dryness, and postoperative radiography revealed unobstructed systems.[7]

In conclusion, many institutions have successfully performed LRC, although oncologic follow-up is relatively short and published patient numbers are few. Many variations of urinary diversion have been described; as groups increase their experience, more purely laparoscopic techniques will be used successfully.

INDICATIONS AND CONTRAINDICATIONS

Indications for LRC mirror those for open radical cystectomy: tumor invading the muscularis propria, high-grade or invasive tumors associated with carcinoma in situ, carcinoma in situ resistant to intravesical therapies, or recurrent, bulky, or symptomatic superficial tumors.[1] Cystectomy has also been performed for noncancerous causes such as chronic pyocystis, intractable pelvic/bladder pain, interstitial cystitis, or hemorrhagic cystitis.

Absolute contraindications to LRC include severe coagulopathy and active intra-abdominal or urinary infection. Relative contraindications include those common to other laparoscopic procedures, namely, severe cardiopulmonary disease, chronic obstructive pulmonary disease (COPD), obesity, and multiple previous intra-abdominal procedures. Clinicians early in their learning curve must be extremely selective and avoid patients with any of the above issues. With more experience, laparoscopic surgeons can perform this procedure with fewer restrictions on patient selection. Currently, even the most experienced laparoscopists require 7 hours or longer to perform complete LRC with urinary diversion. Moreover, for much of this time the patient remains in steep Trendelenburg position. The prolonged pneumoperitoneum is of concern for patients with

COPD because they have decreased ability to release CO_2, resulting in hypercapnea, hypercarbia, acidosis, and the potential for cardiac arrhythmias. Furthermore, prolonged Trendelenburg position negatively affects the anesthesiologist's ability to ventilate the patient due to increased diaphragmatic pressure on the pleural cavity.

In regard to obese patients, simply establishing laparoscopic access can be technically challenging. Moreover, long instruments may be required to safely reach the pelvis. Creation of an ileal loop diversion in overweight patients can be problematic due to the relatively short bowel mesentery compared with a thick abdominal wall. Large amounts of intra-abdominal fat may also make dissection and exposure more difficult. For these reasons, extensive experience with laparoscopy and open surgery in obese patients is recommended before this undertaking.

Previous intra-abdominal procedures can create bowel adhesions and increase the risk of bowel injury. Use extreme care when inserting trocars to avoid inadvertent bowel injury. With experience, bowel adhesions can be mobilized readily using sharp dissection without cautery, usually allowing a straightforward procedure.

In summary, until the surgeon becomes very confident with this procedure, patients should be thin, have had no previous intra-abdominal surgery, and not have obvious bulky disease. Patients with one or more contraindications may nevertheless be considered possible candidates for LRC followed by open creation of urinary diversion.

PATIENT PREOPERATIVE EVALUATION AND PREPARATION

Before radical cystectomy, patients undergo evaluation to rule out metastatic disease. Axial imaging by computed tomography (CT) or magnetic resonance imaging (MRI) with contrast is recommended to assess for tumor bulk, local extension, regional and distant lymphadenopathy, and distant metastasis. Chest, abdominal, and pelvic imaging are recommended, although for lower-stage disease, a chest radiograph rather than CT or MRI should suffice. Bone scans have not proved necessary and are reserved for patients with bony symptoms or significantly elevated alkaline phosphatase. A bimanual examination is also recommended to better estimate residual tumor bulk following transurethral resection because large tumor bulk or questionably fixed disease makes laparoscopic cystectomy significantly more challenging and indicates a poorer prognosis.

Before laparoscopic cystectomy, adequate mechanical and antibiotic bowel preparation are recommended. Marking for an ileal conduit by an enterostomal therapist is also recommended regardless of the diversion entertained in case of inability to perform continent diversion for whatever reason. Prophylactic anticoagulation is strongly considered. General anesthesia with or without regional anesthesia for added intraoperative and postoperative pain management is recommended.

OPERATING ROOM CONFIGURATION AND PATIENT POSITIONING

The room is set-up so that both surgeon and assistants can see the operative field easily (Fig. 25–1). Because these are lengthy procedures, the monitors, one on each side, are set up at the proper height to minimize neck strain and also angled so that personnel will not have to crane their necks to see them. A right-handed surgeon typically stands on the left side with an assistant on the right side. The scrub nurse is also on the right closer to the patient's feet. A monitor is between the first assistant and the scrub nurse (for the surgeon) and one is on the other side for the assistant and nurse. An accessory monitor for others watching the procedure away from the operative field can be set up as well. All instrument trays are kept at the foot of the bed and to the right of the scrub nurse.

Place the patient supine with arms adducted, with all pressure points well padded, on an electric operative table. The frog-leg position is adequate for male patients unless total urethrectomy is planned, in which case a low modified lithotomy with stirrups is used. Place female patients in low modified lithotomy as well, with Yellowfins or comparable stirrups that allow for easy access to both perineum and abdomen. If used, the Automated Endoscopic System for Optimal Positioning (AESOP) robotic camera-holder (Intuitive Surgical, Sunnyvale, CA) is fastened to the operating room table on the right side just lateral to the right shoulder. Then secure the patient to the operative table with heavy, wide tape strips (over towels) placed over legs, thighs, and upper chest, such that there is no patient movement during Trendelenburg or airplaning of the table intraoperatively. Once the patient is prepped and draped, insert a sterile Foley catheter.

TROCAR PLACEMENT

A five-port approach is used (Fig. 25–2). Insufflate the abdoment via the superior aspect of the umbilicus with a Veress needle to establish pneumoperitoneum. Once 15-mm pressure is reached, make a 12-mm incision just above the umbilicus (to stay above the urachus), and place a 10/12-mm trocar through it using a Visiport (U.S. Surgical, Norwalk, CT). Subsequently use direct visualization to place the other ports. Two 10/12-mm ports are a necessary minimum: the initial one for the camera at the umbilicus, and one for the main working port lateral to the right rectus muscle at the level of the umbilicus. The 10/12-mm ports are required for easy use of the endo-GIA stapler, and most surgeons prefer having another 12-mm port (rather than a 5-mm port) on the left side as well, for the flexibility of using of an endo-GIA or 10-mm clip applier on that side. Two more ports are routinely placed: a 5-mm port superomedial to the anterior superior iliac spine on the right (for the assistant), and another in mirror-image location on the left side (for retraction of structures by the surgeon and/or second assistant if available), taking care to avoid the epigastric vessels (Fig. 25–3). Retraction through such a port by the surgeon can be done with a locking grasper that is then fixed to the drapes by pulling the drape through the instrument handle and clamping the drape and instrument in position with a Kelly clamp or similar instrument.

PROCEDURE

Pelvic Lymphadenectomy

Place the patient in modest Trendelenburg slightly airplaned toward the surgeon. For most cases, use the right and left ports

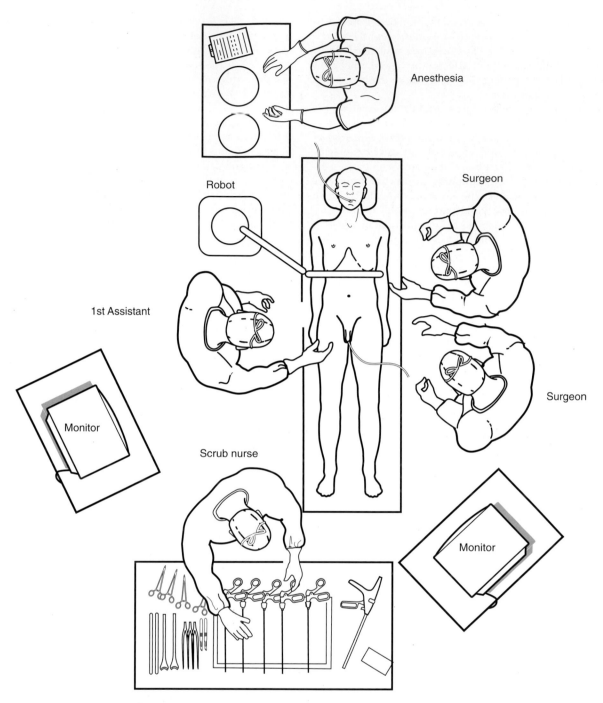

FIGURE 25–1. Operating room setup. The surgeon is typically on the left side, and the first assistant and camera-holding robot are on the right. Each gets a dedicated monitor, unless a large screen is available at the foot of the bed.

that most closely flank the umbilicus. With an alligator grasper in the left hand and a working tool in the right hand (our preference is the Harmonic ACE ultrasonic instrument [Ethicon Endo-Surgery, Cincinnati, OH]), inspect the abdomen for carcinomatosis. If the decision is made to proceed, incise the parietal peritoneum over the vasa deferentia as they cross over the median umbilical ligament (Fig. 25–4).

In men, clip and cut the vasa because they are the median umbilical ligaments, allowing optimal exposure of the pelvic lymph node beds and the posterolateral bladder pedicles (Fig. 25–5). Perform bilateral obturator and iliac lymphadenecto-

mies, staying medial to the genitofemoral nerves and inferior to the bifurcation of the iliac arteries, unless a more extended lymphadenectomy is chosen. Extract these lymph node specimens in discrete packets through the 10/12-mm working ports. Use the distal ends of the vasa as guides to identify the tips of the seminal vesicles, which are identified in order to allow for nerve-sparing cystectomy (Fig. 25–6). Finally, join the parietal peritoneum incisions on either side in the midline posterior to the bladder (see Fig. 25–4).

In women, identify the ureters as they cross over the iliac arteries, and dissect the pelvic lymph node packets identically.

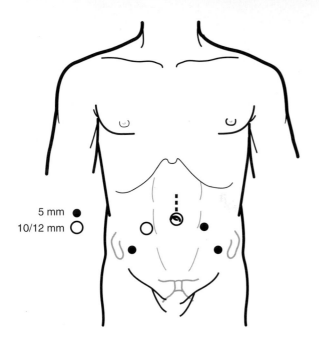

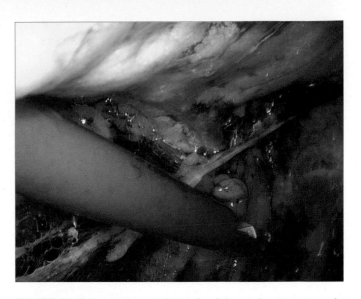

FIGURE 25–3. Ports may require being placed close to the epigastric vessels, which fortunately can be well visualized in some patients and carefully avoided.

FIGURE 25–2. Port placement. At least two 10/12-mm ports should be used, one for a camera and one for needle, Endo-GIA stapler, and other large-bore instrument insertion. The other three ports can be 5-mm ports.

5 mm ●
10/12 mm ○

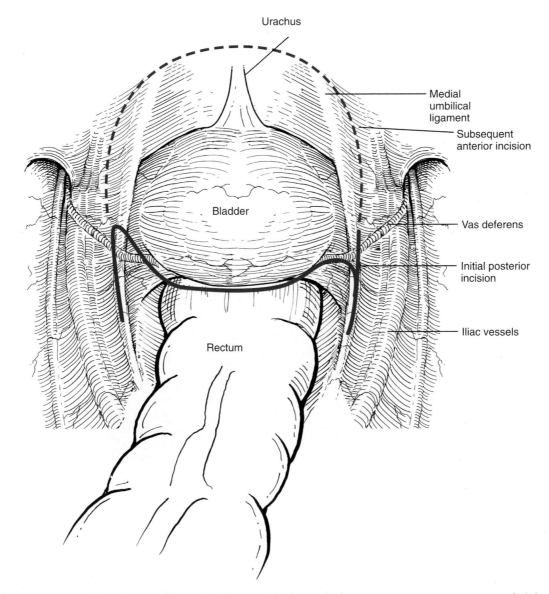

FIGURE 25–4. Peritoneal incision lines. These can be made with a cautery hook or with ultrasonic shears. They are necessary to find the vasa deferentia, dissect posteriorly, and then dissect anteriorly.

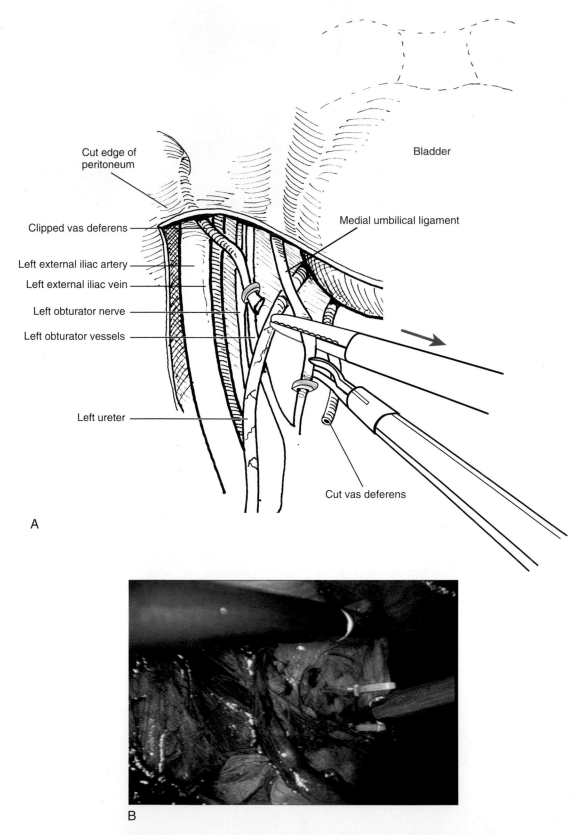

Cut edge of
peritoneum

Bladder

Clipped vas deferens

Medial umbilical ligament

Left external iliac artery

Left external iliac vein

Left obturator nerve

Left obturator vessels

Left ureter

Cut vas deferens

A

B

FIGURE 25–5. *A,* Exposing left posterior bladder. An alligator forceps is being used to retract the left medial umbilical ligament, which has been clipped and is being cut. This maneuver exposes the external iliac vein to help initiate pelvic lymphadenectomy. *B,* To initiate the left pelvic lymphadenectomy, the left medial umbilical ligament is being retracted medially to expose the left external iliac vein. The left vas deferens has already been transected, and the medial umbilical ligament is now being clipped and cut.

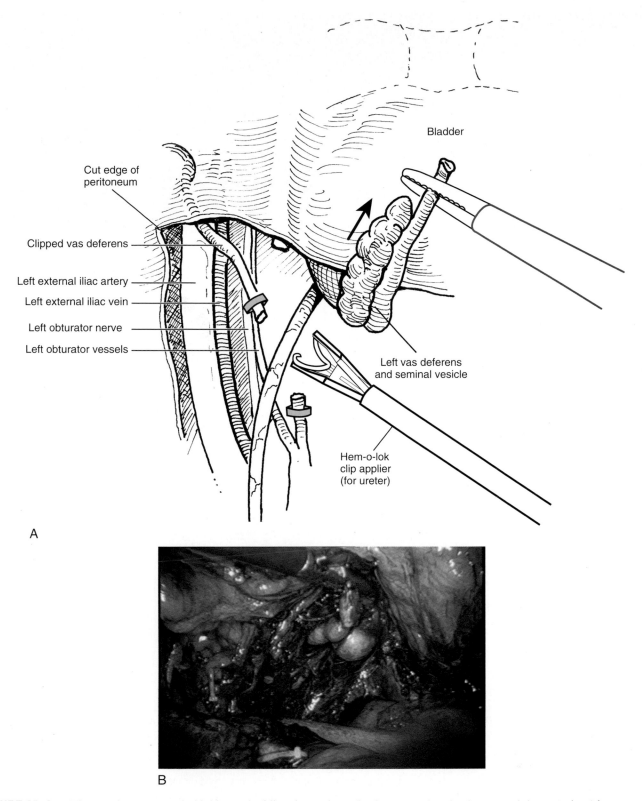

FIGURE 25–6. *A,* The ureter's course into the bladder can be followed once the vas has been cut and its distal stump and the seminal vesicle are retracted superomedially. *B,* The distal left vas deferens (specimen side) is being retracted superomedially to identify the left seminal vesicle for nerve-sparing dissection.

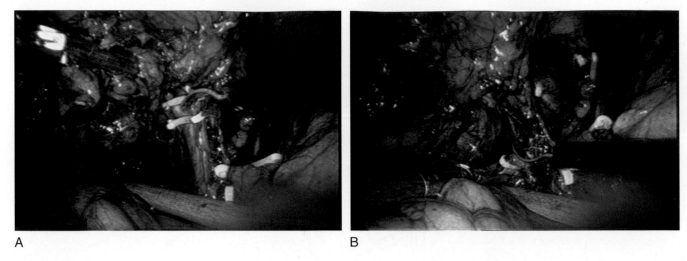

A   B

FIGURE 25–7. *A*, The right ureter is being clipped and cut. The distal cut end of the right vas deferens is being held for medial retraction, exposing the right seminal vesicle tip and the right ureter. *B*, The proximal end of the right ureter is being held up and a distal margin is being taken with scissors for frozen section analysis.

Taking the medial umbilical ligaments can also facilitate the lymph node dissection.

Ureters

Identify the ureters as they cross over the iliac arteries and dive inferiorly into the pelvis. More distally, they lie just lateral to the seminal vesicles in men (Figs. 25–6*A* and 25–7*A*). Once identified and followed toward the bladder in patients of either gender, take the ureters about 2 cm from their vesical insertion (see Fig. 25–7*A*), clip them, and send a frozen section of each distal ureter for pathologic analysis (see Fig. 25–7*B*).

Posterior Dissection

In men, incise Denonvillier's fascia in the posterior midline just inferior to the prostatic midline where the seminal vesicles insert. It may help to retract the sigmoid posterosuperiorly and the bladder superiorly. Identify the plane between the rectum and posterior prostate and develop it bluntly. Lateral to it, the vascular pedicles to the bladder come into view. Retracting a seminal vesicle tip medially and superiorly and working laterally to this, take one and then the other pedicle with roticulating endo-GIA staplers (2- to 2.5-mm clips, 4.5-cm length) (Fig. 25–8). Typically, two in-line firings are needed on each side (Fig. 25–9).

In women, retract the uterus anteriorly and the sigmoid posterosuperiorly as necessary, and use an endo-GIA stapler to transect the infundibulosuspensory ligaments. Taking these ligaments with their associated ovarian vasculature allows anterior retraction of the adnexal structures and exposure of the peritoneum overlying the posterior vaginal fornix. This can be identified by a sponge stick in the vagina or, as recently demonstrated by Moinzadeh and colleagues,[10] using a Koh cervical cup and Rumi manipulator (Cooper Surgical, Shelton, CT). Gently score the parietal peritoneum here with electrocautery, and turn attention anterolaterally at this point.

Anterior Dissection

In men, the final firings of the endo-GIA lead one to the prostatic pedicles. At this point, proceed to the anterior dissection, which is accomplished via a parietal peritoneal inverted-U–shaped incision incorporating the urachus and bladder that connects with the peritoneotomy made for the posterior dissection (see Fig. 25–4). This can be facilitated by instilling 120 mL of saline in the bladder temporarily. Then drop the bladder, define the space of Retzius, and expose the puboprostatic ligaments. Incise the endopelvic fasciae and puboprostatic ligaments, and place and tie a dorsal vein stitch (2-0 Vicryl, GS-21 needle) (Fig. 25–10). Cut the dorsal vein using an electrocautery hook, ultrasonic shears, or an endo-GIA stapler, and expose the urethra. At this point, cut the urethra with scissors, leaving just enough of a stump to clip with a 10-mm Hem-o-lok (Weck Closure Systems, Research Triangle Park, NC) in order to prevent urine spillage (Fig. 25–11). Typically, send a distal margin for frozen section, and remove the catheter. Sharply incise the posterior striated sphincter, and then perform retrograde dissection of the prostatic pedicles, with nerve-sparing possible as clinically indicated (Fig. 25–12).

In women, drop the bladder in similar fashion, until the bladder pedicles come into view. Remember to empty the bladder of any instilled saline, then grasp detrusor muscle near the clipped distal ureteral stumps and retract superomedially. As the assistant provides inferolateral countertraction on the pelvic floor, the pedicles come into view. Again, two firings of a roticulating endo-GIA stapler (2- to 2.5-mm clips, 4.5-cm length) are usually adequate for each pedicle. At this point, proceed anteriorly to the midline, retracting both uterus and bladder inferiorly and exposing the endopelvic fascia and dorsal vein. Work here just as in men, incising the fasciae and controlling the dorsal vein. Then move posteriorly again and cut through the posterior fornix in the midline onto a sponge stick or onto the Koh cervical ring. Extend this incision into the vagina on both sides distally to the vaginal outlet, typically excising the anterior third of the vagina as a strip en bloc with the posterior bladder. One way to prevent loss of pneumoperi-

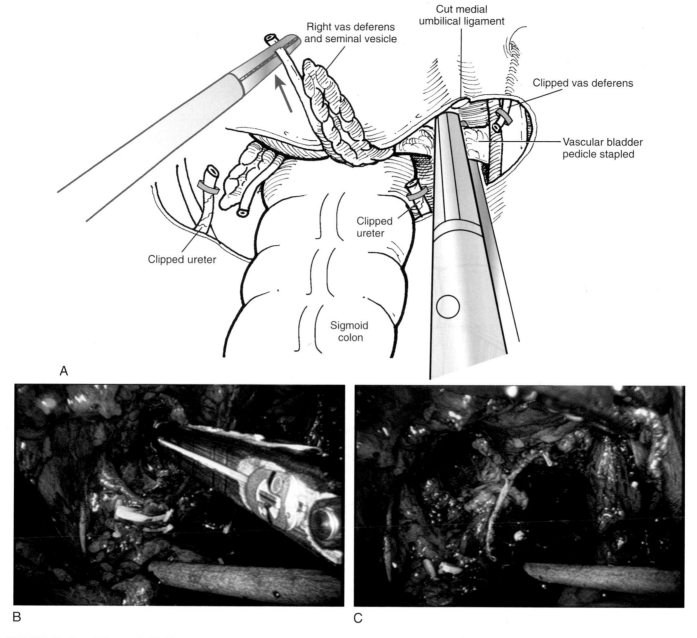

FIGURE 25–8. *A,* Taking right bladder pedicle. Once the ureters have been transected, the vascular bladder pedicles can be taken with roticulating Endo-GIA stapling devices as the vas/seminal vesicle complexes are retracted superomedially. *B,* The left pedicle is being taken with a roticulating Endo-GIA stapling device (2.5-mm clips). *C,* The Endo-GIA stapler has been fired once and the first clip line is seen at the left pedicle.

toneum is to occlude the vagina with a wet laparotomy pad placed in a surgical glove, and apply this to the vaginal vault. However, the insufflation balloon that is a part of the Koh colpotomizer system is quite effective for this purpose.

Specimen Extraction

In men, once the retrograde dissection lines meet the endo-GIA pedicle clips, clip and cut final attachments with Hem-o-lok clips, freeing up the specimen. Place the specimen into a 15-mm EndoCatch (U.S. Surgical) impermeable bag and cinch it shut (Fig. 25–13). Specimen extraction is typically done via a lower midline incision, which is then used for extracorporeal creation of the urinary diversion, although specimen extraction can also be performed through an enlarged subsequent ileal conduit stoma site, and even rectum (before rectosigmoid pouch creation). If urethrectomy is indicated, it may proceed once the specimen is extracted.

In women, handle the urethra as in the previous section if orthotopic diversion is planned. Alternately, if total en bloc urethrectomy is planned, do not cut the urethra during the anterior dissection but instead core it out perineally with electrocautery along with the anterior vaginal wall. Once freed up, extract the specimen transvaginally, then perform laparoscopic vaginal reconstruction (usually a running 2-0 Vicryl stitch is

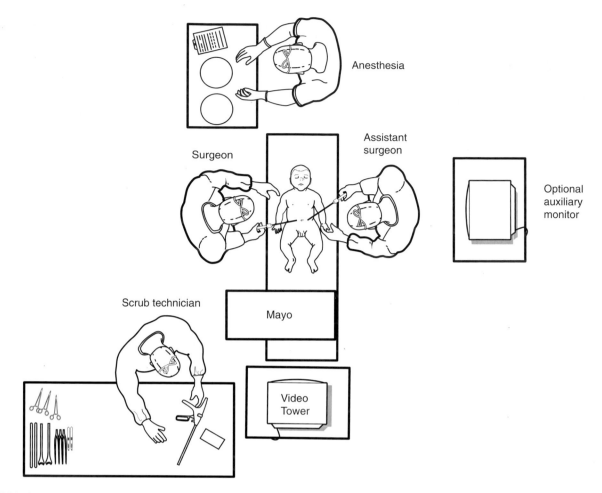

FIGURE 26–1. Operating room configuration. The monitor is placed at the foot of the bed to allow adequate visualization of the pelvis for the entire surgical team. The surgeon stands contralateral to the affected testis with an auxiliary slave monitor placed across the table for the primary surgeon.

OPERATING ROOM CONFIGURATION AND PATIENT POSITIONING

The operating room configuration includes one monitor at the foot of the bed to allow adequate visualization of the pelvis by all members of the surgical team (Fig. 26–1). Stand on the side contralateral to the affected testis. An auxiliary slave monitor may be placed across the table from the primary surgeon; however, when operating in the deep pelvis, we have found the monitor at the foot of the bed to be more ergonomic.

After induction of general endotracheal anesthesia, administer prophylactic broad-spectrum antibiotics and place a grounding pad. Leave the child supine with the legs parted moderately or frog-legged. Repeat examination of the groin under anesthesia may identify a testis and obviate the need for laparoscopic evaluation. Pad all pressure points without elevating the extremities to an extent that will compromise exposure to the scrotum or pelvis. Place a small smooth roll under the sacrum to elevate and open the pelvis, if needed.

Prep and drape the child from the xiphoid to the upper thighs. Use an orogastric tube to decompress gases from a tearful separation and induction of anesthesia. Place a urethral catheter after the sterile prep and leave it indwelling throughout the case.

TROCAR PLACEMENT

Three ports are generally sufficient to complete the procedure, with a rare fourth port needed to retract bowel or other obstructing structure. Place the first trocar in an immediate supraumbilical or infraumbilical position, as described later. Increase the peritoneal pressure temporarily to 20 mm Hg for insertion of additional trocars under direct visualization, if desired. Place the second and third ports, each 3 mm or 5 mm depending on available equipment, at the level of the umbilicus in the mid-clavicular line (Fig. 26–2). The vector of each trocar is toward the affected groin. Take care to avoid the epigastric vessels. Placement of these ports just above the level of the umbilicus instead allows additional room for movement of instruments in the smaller infant. This configuration affords freedom for the surgeon and camera without compromising the triangulation needed for the laparoscopist to work efficiently.

Once optimally positioned, secure each trocar to the a bdominal wall with suture to prevent inadvertent withdrawal during instrument exchange. Trendelenburg positioning with table rotation to the unaffected side will facilitate displacement of the bowel for safe visualization of the anatomy.

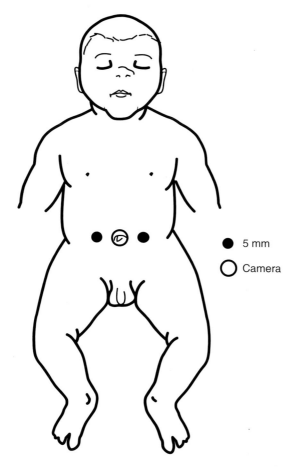

● 5 mm

○ Camera

FIGURE 26–2. Trocar placement. A periumbilical port is initially placed, with second and third ports placed at the level of the umbilicus in the midclavicular line.

PROCEDURE

Diagnostic Laparoscopy

Achieve peritoneal insufflation in children via a small semilunar incision in the infraumbilical or supraumbilical rim or by a transumbilical approach; excellent cosmesis results in each case. Obtain access to the peritoneum via direct blind puncture (Veress needle technique) or open insertion (Hasson trocar technique). Insert the trocar at a 45-degree angle toward the pelvis to minimize the risk of visceral injury. These techniques and respective precautions are described in detail elsewhere in the text, and the approach largely depends on the training and preference of the surgeon. After insertion of a 5-mm umbilical port, perform CO_2 insufflation at low flow to achieve a pressure of 12 mm Hg in infants and 15 mm Hg in the older child. Use disposable or reusable trocars. Radially dilating introducers are also useful for insertion of trocars. Defer placement of additional ports until the gonad is identified and plans for therapeutic laparoscopy are in place.

After safely entering the peritoneal cavity, briefly inspect the abdominal and pelvic contents to rule out injury or obvious coincident pathology. Rare adhesions may be encountered in the pelvis in children with a history of prior abdominal operation or infection. Perform careful dissection with either the EndoShears or ultrasonic dissector to facilitate exposure.

The inguinal ring may be more difficult to see in the child with a high abdominal testis because the anatomic landscape is less populated. The contralateral ring is a useful reference in that situation. The normal inguinal ring is marked by the confluence of the vas deferens (medial) and spermatic vessels (lateral) (Fig. 26–3). Their relationship with the iliacs and ureter, as well as the obliterated umbilical artery and inferior epigastric vessels, is also noteworthy for the progression of the case.

The vas deferens travels in the retroperitoneum in the deep pelvis, crossing the obliterated umbilical artery laterally and the distal ureter medially after exiting the deep inguinal ring. The spermatic vessels come into view from just beneath the ipsilateral colonic peritoneal reflection and follow a retroperitoneal course toward the internal inguinal ring (see Fig. 26–3). The vessels guide the surgeon to the testis, which can be anywhere along the course of normal testicular descent from the renal hilum to the pelvis. Uncommonly, the testis may be found near the liver or spleen, in the deep pelvis behind the bladder, or ectopic in the contralateral hemipelvis. The vas deferens, gonadal vessels, and testis compose a triangle, with the testis at the apex. This triangle serves as the platform for the posterior peritoneal dissection and pedicle mobilization.

Intraoperative Decisions

The next phase of surgical intervention depends on the findings during laparoscopic exploration; potential scenarios are outlined as follows.

1. *An intra-abdominal testis is identified.* If the testis is located near the internal ring or below the level of the iliac vessels, one-stage laparoscopic orchiopexy is appropriate. However, for a very high testis with a short vascular leash, consider a two-stage procedure before extensive dissection (see discussion of two-stage laparoscopic Fowler-Stephens).

2. *A normal vas deferens and spermatic vessels exit the inguinal ring.* If the inguinal ring is closed, explore the groin for a probable vanishing testis. The need for excision of these remnants is controversial but recommended, because the "nubbin" contains viable germ cell elements in 10% of cases.[23,24] If the inguinal ring is open, a "peeping" testis may be located just inside the canal and may be milked into the abdomen for laparoscopic mobilization. Otherwise, perform inguinal exploration.

3. *Blind-ending vas and vessels are identified.* This is the only scenario in which no further exploration is required.

4. *Blind-ending vas is identified.* Further laparoscopic exploration is required to identify the gonadal vessels. Dysjunction can occur between the testis and Wolffian structures; if a testis is present, it will be related to the vessels. Blind-ending vessels are required to terminate exploration.

Components of Laparoscopic Orchiopexy

After peritoneal insufflation and identification of a low intra-abdominal or a "peeping" testis at the internal ring, laparoscopic orchiopexy is completed with the following basic steps:

1. Place trocars (see earlier).
2. Dissect the testis and vascular pedicle.
3. Create the Dartos pouch.

hear failure, pneumonia, ileus, thrombophlebitis, pulmonary embolism, ureteral stent migration, ureteral stent clot obstruction, ureteral edema, urinary leakage, urinoma, anastomotic stricture, and delayed stone formation.[5,7,9]

Tips and Tricks

- For right pyeloplasty, consider placing a working trocar in the midclavicular line in the upper abdomen to have both working trocars in line with the anastomosis for easier suturing.
- Consider additional traction or holding sutures at the apex and at the top of the anastomosis to align the ureter and pelvis for an improved, watertight anastomosis.
- For infant pyeloplasty, place working trocars as far apart as possible to minimize dueling of instruments.

REFERENCES

1. Peters CA: Laparoscopy in pediatric urology. Curr Opin Urol 14:67–73, 2004.
2. Schuessler WW, Grune MT, Tecuanhuey LV, et al: Laparoscopic dismembered pyeloplasty. J Urol 150:695–704, 1993.
3. Peters CA, Schlussel RN, Retik AB: Pediatric laparoscopic dismembered pyeloplasty. J Urol 153:1962–1965, 1995.
4. Adeyoju AB, Hrouda D, Gill IS: Laparoscopic pyeloplasty: The first decade. BJU Int 94:264–267, 2004
5. Munver R, Sosa RE, Del Pizzo JJ: Laparoscopic pyeloplasty: History, evolution, and future. J Endourol 18:748–755, 2004.
6. Olsen LH, Jorgensen TM: Computer assisted pyeloplasty in children: The retroperitoneal approach. J Urol 171:2629–2631, 2004.
7. Inagaki T, Rha KH, Ong AM, et al: Laparoscopic pyeloplasty: Current status. BJU Int 95 (Suppl 2):102–105, 2005.
8. Siu W, Seifman BD, Wolf JS Jr: Subcutaneous emphysema, pneumomediastinum and bilateral pneumothoraces after laparoscopic pyeloplasty. J Urol 170:1936–1937, 2003.
9. Soulie M, Salomon L, Patard JJ, et al: Extraperitoneal laparoscopic pyeloplasty: A multicenter study of 55 procedures. J Urol 166:48–50, 2001.

CHAPTER 28

Complications of Laparoscopic Surgery

Lee Richstone
Louis R. Kavoussi

The benefit of any surgical intervention is weighed against the inevitable risk of complications. Although experience is of obvious importance, not even the most veteran surgeon is immune to complications that may occur during or after an operation. The potential for complications and unexpected events may arise from a multitude of sources, including the individuality of a given patient's anatomy, physiology, or disease. Variations in the operative environment, including staffing, anesthetic, and nursing issues, as well as equipment malfunction, also contribute to outcome. The possibility of a technical misadventure is also a constant risk. When complications do occur, early recognition and aggressive treatment are crucial in order to minimize subsequent morbidity to the patient.

Many of the complications that may occur during laparoscopic retroperitoneal surgery are similar to those encountered with traditional open surgery. However, controlling these events requires a unique skill set. Significant differences in the postoperative presentation of these complications may exist between the laparoscopic and open approaches. Moreover, some complications are unique to laparoscopic surgery. Fortunately, the tremendous growth of laparoscopy has allowed for a better understanding of the potential pitfalls associated with the endoscopic approach. Cumulative experience has helped to better quantify the risks associated with laparoscopy. The lessons learned have led to the formation of defensive strategies for prevention as well as treatment plans to deal with complications once they occur.

Complications from laparoscopic procedures may arise from almost every aspect of the operation, beginning with patient selection and preoperative planning. Once in the operating room, complications may arise from patient positioning, obtaining initial access, trocar placement, the establishment of pneumoperitoneum, dissection, or closure. In this chapter, we review the potential complications that can occur during each of these areas. Strategies aimed at complication prevention, recognition, and treatment are discussed.

PREOPERATIVE PLANNING

Preventing complications begins with careful patient selection and preoperative management. Active infections are treated and any coagulopathies are addressed before laparoscopic surgery is undertaken. Anticoagulant medication is discontinued before surgery. Medical and cardiac clearances are sought when indicated. Patients with significant cardiopulmonary disease may be unable to tolerate pneumoperitoneum and may require use of helium insufflant or conversion to an open procedure. Assessing the level of difficulty and the appropriateness of the laparoscopic approach for a given case is largely dependent on the experience of the surgeon. For example, although a laparoscopic nephrectomy can be successfully performed on an individual with a 15-cm tumor, inexperienced surgeons may not wish to attempt such cases.

Informed Consent and Patient Expectations

Obtaining and documenting appropriate informed consent are critical before initiating any surgical procedure and has particular relevance should a complication arise. Although no patient wishes to believe that he or she will have a suboptimal outcome, it is important to review the potential complications of a given laparoscopic procedure to ensure that the patient has reasonable expectations. Many patients mistakenly equate the smaller scars and diminished pain of laparoscopy with lesser risk. A significant learning curve exists for many laparoscopic procedures, and the surgeon's personal experience and complication rates should be discussed. Although laparoscopic renal surgery is less morbid than comparable open approaches, many patients assume that their postoperative course will be similar to that seen with other commonly performed laparoscopic procedures, such as tubal ligation and cholecystectomy. The surgeon must explain that laparoscopic renal surgery is associated with more postoperative discomfort than some of the more commonly performed laparoscopic procedures. Patients must always be made aware that conversion to an open procedure may be necessary to safely complete the proposed operation. Discussion of this point takes psychological pressure off the surgeon to try to complete the operation laparoscopically if circumstances may be more optimally handled by an open procedure.

Radiographic Planning

Preoperative imaging is essential to aid in surgical planning, access, and dissection and to help avoid complications. Computed tomography with three-dimensional reconstruction may be of value in assessing the anatomy of the renal vasculature, collecting system, and parenchyma during partial nephrectomy and living donor nephrectomy. Imaging studies that answer all relevant anatomic questions should be obtained and readily available in the operative suite. Once the patient is on the operative table, inspection of the surface anatomy relative to the radiographs will aid in optimal port placement.

Anesthetic Concerns

The physiologic impact of a moderate (10–20 mm Hg) CO_2 pneumoperitoneum is manifold, with significant effects on the

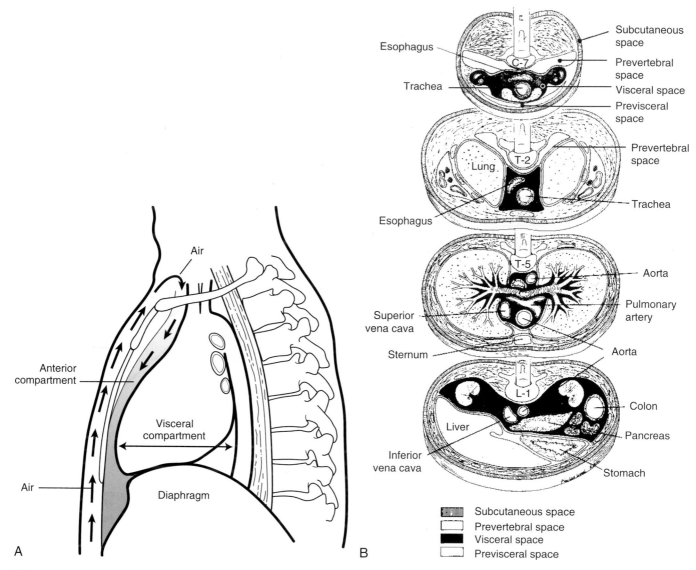

FIGURE 28–6. *A,* Anatomic fascial planes in the neck communicate with the subcutaneous tissue planes allowing for egress of gas into the mediastinum. *B,* Compartments of the mediastinum. The viscera of middle compartment are in continuity with the neck and retroperitoneum.

is usually of no clinical consequence; once the procedure is complete, the gas is absorbed. However, extensive dissection of gas can lead to pneumothorax, pneumomediastinum, and hypercarbia. The risk of development of a pneumomediastinum increases when crepitus is noted extending up to the neck. Due to a continuum of fascial planes existing between the cervical soft tissue and mediastinum, the potential exists for gas to track upward into the neck and down into the mediastinum[35,36] (Fig. 28–6). Subclinical thoracic air collections have been reported in 5.5% of urologic laparoscopic procedures, which can often be managed conservatively due to the high solubility of CO_2.[37,38] However, if symptomatic pneumothorax or pneumomediastinum develops, the pneumoperitoneum should be discontinued and the ectopic gas evacuated.

A pneumothorax can also occur in the absence of subcutaneous emphysema. Insufflant can enter the pleural space through anatomic or congenital defects in the diaphragm. Complica-

tions of anesthesia and positive-pressure ventilation, as well as patient conditions such as emphysematous bullae, can also lead to the entry of air into the pleural cavity.[39]

After the pneumoperitoneum is successfully established, the presence of pressurized gas in the abdominal cavity has significant and variegated physiologic consequences that can result in complications. The cumulative response of the cardiovascular system during laparoscopy with CO_2 under moderate pressure (10–20 mm Hg) is generally sufficient for healthy individuals to tolerate pneumoperitoneum. However, patients with significant cardiovascular or pulmonary disease may not compensate sufficiently. In addition, careful attention to insufflation pressure is critical to avoid excessive tension and potential cardiovascular collapse.

Although appropriate ventilatory adjustments are usually sufficient to eliminate the increased CO_2 load that results from laparoscopy, in some patients, CO_2 insufflation can produce

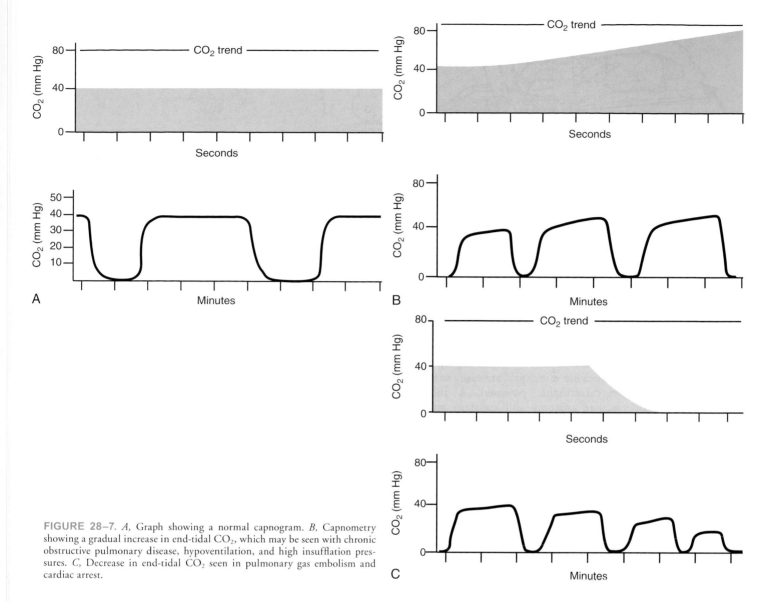

FIGURE 28–7. *A,* Graph showing a normal capnogram. *B,* Capnometry showing a gradual increase in end-tidal CO_2, which may be seen with chronic obstructive pulmonary disease, hypoventilation, and high insufflation pressures. *C,* Decrease in end-tidal CO_2 seen in pulmonary gas embolism and cardiac arrest.

profound hypercapnia. This can be exacerbated by subcutaneous emphysema and excessive intra-abdominal pressures. If severe, hypercapnia and acidosis can have significant depressive cardiac effects. Initial management consists of lowering the intra-abdominal pressure. If the anesthesiologist cannot adequately compensate, helium may be used or the procedure may need to be converted to open surgery.

Insufflation can also produce significant cardiac arrhythmias, including bradycardia, tachycardia, ventricular extrasystoles, atrioventricular dissociation, and nodal rhythms. Hypercapnia, as well as a vagal response to abdominal distention and peritoneal irritation, has been implicated. The use of atropine prior to insufflation may prevent these vagal reactions.[40]

A rare but potentially fatal complication related to the pneumoperitoneum is a gas embolism, which occurs most commonly during the induction of pneumoperitoneum. Although intravasation of gas due to the increased intra-abdominal pressure has been suggested as an etiology, the most common cause is direct placement of a needle or trocar into a vessel or abdominal organ.[41,42] In a meta-analysis of nearly 500,000 laparoscopic procedures with closed access, the incidence of gas emboli was 0.0014%.[43]

Patient survival after gas embolism depends on rapid diagnosis and treatment. The diagnosis can be difficult, and there is often no warning before acute cardiovascular collapse, particularly during insufflation. When the size of the embolus increases, tachycardia, arrhythmias, hypotension, and increased central venous pressure may be noted. Hypoxia, hypercapnia, and cyanosis may also be evident. Electrocardiographic changes can include a right heart strain pattern, and auscultation may reveal the classic "mill wheel" murmur just before the acute event. Also, an acute decrease in measured end-tidal CO_2 measurements is noted as the embolism occludes the pulmonary trunk (Fig. 28–7). When an embolism is suspected, release the pneumoperitoneum and administer 100% oxygen. Place the patient in the left lateral decubitus position with the head down to move the gas away from the pulmonary artery (Fig. 28–8). Institute cardiopulmonary resuscitation, and place a central venous catheter in an attempt to aspirate the gas. Percutaneous or open evacuation of the gas may be indicated.[44–47]

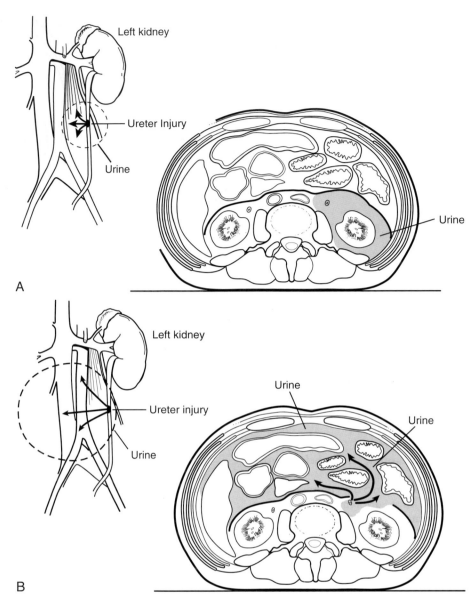

FIGURE 28–18. *A,* Ureteral injury can result in the development of a large retroperitoneal urinoma. *B,* If the peritoneum is not intact, peritonitis can result from seepage of urine and subsequent bowel irritation.

complications can be classified as intraoperative (3.5%–8%), postoperative (1.8%–2%), or delayed (4%).[55,56,58] Hemorrhage associated with LPN can occur during tumor resection due to inadequate hilar clamping or on revascularization secondary to insufficient hemostatic control of the resection bed.[55] Successful identification of supernumerary renal arteries and correct placement of laparoscopic bulldog or Satinsky clamps are critical to ensure hilar control. Although performing LPN without hilar clamping has been reported, it is associated with increased blood loss and limits the clear visualization of renal parenchyma necessary for identifying the renal mass and ensuring surgical margins.[59] Proficient intracorporeal suturing skills are prerequisite for control of parenchymal bleeding and renorrhaphy. Bioadhesives and sealants are useful adjuncts and may reduce hemorrhagic complications during LPN.[60]

Urinary leakage is a well-recognized complication after nephron-sparing surgery. In open series, urinary leak is a common postoperative complication, seen in 1.4% to 17.4% of patients.[61,62] In LPN series, urinary leak ranges from 1.4% to 10%.[55-58] Intraoperative identification of collecting system entry and suture repair of the collecting system may avoid leakage.

In an attempt to reduce urinary fistula formation, some surgeons advocate the placement of an ipsilateral ureteral catheter before nephron-sparing surgery, allowing for retrograde dye injection as an aid to identify entry into the collecting system.[63] However, the use of this approach is controversial, and some authors have reported that ureteral stent placement does not reduce the incidence of early or delayed urinary leaks.[64] Tumor location and size, as well as the experience of the surgeon, should guide the decision of whether to perform retrograde injection of dye during LPN. It must be noted, however, that even with visualization and repair of collecting system entry, urinary leakage can still occur.

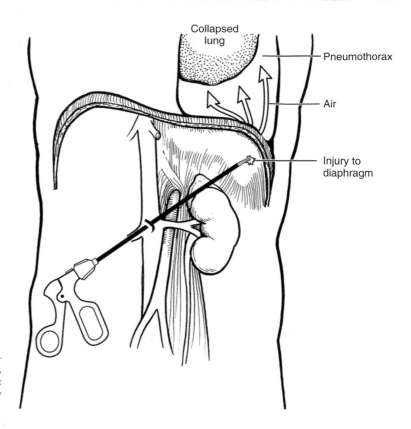

FIGURE 28–19. Injury to the diaphragm can occur during aggressive lateral dissection of the upper pole of the kidney, adrenal gland, or spleen. This injury is usually immediately apparent as the patient will rapidly show signs of increased peak airway pressures, difficulty with ventilation, and, if not corrected, tension pneumothorax.

Coagulation necrosis secondary to excessive electrocautery may contribute to urinary leakage.[65] Therefore, after the use of monopolar electrocautery to outline the circumferential margin of resection, many authors advocate the use of "cold" laparoscopic scissors to perform the resection in attempt to reduce coagulation necrosis and the risk of urinary leak.[64]

Operative treatment for urinary fistula is rarely needed following LPN. Resolution can be expected with conservative management involving the use of prolonged suction drainage. Ureteral stent placement or percutaneous nephrostomy drainage is rarely needed.

Herniation

Port site hernias are generally uncommon, with an incidence of less than 0.1%.[66] Because hernias are more likely to occur with larger trocars, attempt to close them when using ports greater than 10 mm placed anterior to the posterior axillary line. Herniation of bowel into the preperitoneal space (through a peritoneal defect with intact fascia) can occur. Therefore, attempt to close the peritoneum as well as the fascia. Incisional hernias at hand-port sites following hand-assisted laparoscopy have also been reported with an incidence of 1.9%.[67] Take care when using a balloon device to create a working space in the retroperitoneum. If the balloon is inadvertently inflated within the fascia of the abdominal wall, a large defect may be created, resulting in hernia formation. Close all holes in mesentery to avoid a mesenteric hernia.

Laparoscopic Exit

After successful completion of the laparoscopic dissection, it is crucial to maintain vigilance to avoid postoperative problems. It is easy to let down one's guard after the goal of the surgery has been reached following hours of intense concentration. Several set maneuvers must be followed to minimize postoperative pain and the possibility of morbidity.

1. Undertake a thorough examination of the operative field and any ligated vessels to ensure hemostasis. The pneumoperitoneum may have been sufficient to tamponade venous bleeding; therefore, the intra-abdominal pressure should be lowered for 5 minutes, followed by a second inspection. If seepage of blood is noted, patience is crucial in order to locate small bleeding sites. Use electrocautery, suture, or clips as indicated.
2. Once comfortable that hemostasis is complete, survey the bowel and other intra-abdominal structures for injury. Inspect the abdominal cavity for any enteric content emanating from an unrecognized injury. Also, attempt to remove any clots from the abdomen to minimize the risk of postoperative adhesion formation.
3. Perform trocar removal and closure under direct vision. Trocars may tamponade bleeding caused by injury to abdominal wall vessels. Carefully inspect the internal abdominal wall to assess for bleeding or a hematoma after removal of the trocars. If bleeding is noted, perform cautery of the tract or placement of a figure-of-eight suture under direct vision, as needed. If bleeding is significant, place a Foley catheter through the site, inflate it with 20 mL of water, and place it on traction while considering the optimal method of control. A cutdown with open surgical repair may be indicated.
4. In adults, close 10-mm trocar sites anterior to the posterior axillary line to avoid hernia formation. In children, close all 5-mm sites. Close trocar sites under direct vision to minimize the potential for inadvertent bowel injury.

5. Attempt to evacuate all the CO_2 from the abdomen before removal of the last trocar. CO_2 can act as a diaphragmatic irritant, resulting in postoperative back, shoulder, or chest pain. Open the stopcock on the last remaining port with the laparoscope inside. Use the laparoscope to aim the trocar at anterior pockets of gas. The anesthesiologist manually ventilates the patient with large breaths to help with the egress of gas. Once all gas is removed, back the trocar off the laparoscope. Then slowly back the laparoscope out of the trocar site to allow for inspection for bleeding and to prevent evisceration of abdominal content into the tract.
6. Irrigate all sites and inspect them for subcutaneous bleeding to prevent potential infection or hematoma formation. Close the skin and apply the dressing according to preference.

SUMMARY

Complications are an inevitable part of surgical practice. With experience, the overall risks of laparoscopic surgery are equivalent to those seen with open surgical approaches. Laparoscopic renal surgery has well-defined potential risks that need to be discussed in detail with patients. In order to prevent, recognize, and treat complications, the laparoscopist must be thoroughly versed in the potential pitfalls that exist from preoperative planning to laparoscopic exit. Experience and attention to detail can help keep complication rates and patient morbidity to a minimum.

REFERENCES

Anesthetic Concerns

1. Sheinin B, Lindgren L, Scheinin TM: Preoperative nitrous oxide delays bowel function after colonic surgery. Br J Anaesth 64:154, 1990.
2. Taylor E, Reinstein R, White PF, Soper N: Anesthesia for laparoscopic cholecystectomy: Is nitrous oxide contraindicated? Anesthesiology 76:541, 1992.
3. Krogh B, Jorn Jensen P, Henneberg SW, et al: Nitrous oxide does not influence operating conditions or postoperative course in colonic surgery. Br J Anaesth 72:55, 1994.
4. Akca O, Lenhardt R, Fleischmann E, et al: Nitrous oxide increases the incidence of bowel distention in patients undergoing elective colon resection. Acta Anaesthesiol Scand 48:894, 2004.
5. Chiu AW, Chang LS, Birkett DH, Babayan RK: The impact of pneumoperitoneum, pneumoretroperitoneum, and gasless laparoscopy on the systemic and renal hemodynamics. J Am Coll Surg 181:397, 1995.
6. McDougall EM, Monk TG, Wolf JS, et al: The effect of prolonged pneumoperitoneum on renal function in an animal model. J Am Coll Surg 182:317, 1996.

Obesity

7. Mendoza D, Newman R, Albala D, et al: Laparoscopic complication in markedly obese urologic patients: A multi-institutional review. Urology 48:562, 1996.
8. Gill I, Kavoussi LR, Clayman R, et al: Complications of laparoscopic nephrectomy in 185 patients: A multi-institutional review. J Urol 154:479, 1995.
9. Fugita OEH, Chan DY, Roberts WW, et al: Laparoscopic radical nephrectomy in obese patients: Outcomes and technical considerations. Urology 63:247, 2004.
10. Kuo PC, Plotkin JS, Stevens S, et al: Outcomes of laparoscopic donor nephrectomy in obese patients. Transplantation 69:180, 2000.
11. Doublet J, Belair G: Retroperitoneal laparoscopic nephrectomy is safe and effective in obese patients: A comparative study of 55 procedures. Urology 56:63, 2000.
12. Fazeli-Matin S, Gill IS, Hsu THS, et al: Laparoscopic renal and adrenal surgery in obese patients: Comparison to open surgery. J Urol 162:665, 1999.

13. Anast JW, Stoller ML, Meng MV, et al: Differences in complications and outcomes for obese patients undergoing laparoscopic radical, partial or simple nephrectomy. J Urol 172:2287, 2004.

Surgical History

14. Parsons JK, Jarrett TJ, Chow GK, Kavoussi LR: The effect of previous abdominal surgery on urological laparoscopy. J Urol 168:2387, 2002.

The Approach: Retroperitoneal Versus Transperitoneal

15. Desai MM, Strzempkowski B, Matin SF, et al: Prospective randomized comparison of transperitoneal versus retroperitoneal laparoscopic radical nephrectomy. J Urol 173:38, 2000.
16. McDougall EM, Clayman RV: Laparoscopic nephrectomy for benign disease: Comparison of transperitoneal and retroperitoneal approaches. J Endourol 10:45, 1996.
17. Desai MM, Strzempkowski B, Matin SF, et al: Prospective randomized comparison of transperitoneal versus retroperitoneal laparoscopic radical nephrectomy. J Urol 173:38, 2005.
18. Nambirajan, T, Jeschke, S, Al-Zahrani, V, et al: Prospective, randomized controlled study: Transperitoneal versus retroperitoneoscopic radical nephrectomy. Urology 64:919, 2004.
19. Meraney AM, Samee AA-E, Gill IS: Vascular and bowel complications during retroperitoneal laparoscopic surgery. J Urol 168:1941, 2002.

Patient Positioning and Neuromuscular Injuries

20. Wolf JS, Marcovich R, Gill IS, et al: Survey of neuromuscular injuries to the patient and surgeon during urologic laparoscopic surgery. Urology 55:831, 2000.
21. Stevens J, Nicholson E, Linehan WM, et al: Risk factors for skin breakdown after renal and adrenal surgery. Urology 64:246, 2004.

Access and Trocar Placement

22. Catarci M, Carlini M, Gentileschi P, Santoro EL: Major and minor injuries during the creation of pneumoperitoneum. A multicenter study on 12,919 cases. Surg Endosc 15:566, 2001.
23. Bonjer HJ, Hazebroek EJ, Kazemier G, et al: Open versus closed establishment of pneumoperitoneum in laparoscopic surgery. Br J Surg 84:599, 1997.
24. Saville LE, Woods MS: Laparoscopy and major retroperitoneal vascular injuries (MRVI). Surg Endosc 9:1096, 1995.
25. Schafer M, Lauper M, Krahenbuhl L: Trocar and Veress needle injuries during laparoscopy. Surg Endosc 15:275, 2001.
26. Hanney R, Alle K, Cregan P: Major vascular injury and laparoscopy. Aust N Z J Surg 65:533, 1995.
27. Sadeghi-Nejad H, Kavoussi LR, Peters CA: Bowel injury in open technique laparoscopic cannula placement. Urology 43:559, 1994.
28. Woolcott R: The safety of laparoscopy performed by direct trocar insertion and carbon dioxide insufflation under vision. Aust N Z J Obstet Gynaecol 37:216, 1997.
29. String A, Berber E, Foroutani A, et al: Use of the optical access trocar for safe and rapid entry in various laparoscopic procedures. Surg Endosc 15:570, 2001.
30. Thomas MA, Rha KH, Ong AM, et al: Optical access trocar injuries in urological laparoscopic surgery. J Urol 170:61, 2003.
31. Agresta F, DeSimone P, Ciardo LF, Bedlin N: Direct trocar insertion vs Veress needle in nonobese patients undergoing laparoscopic procedures. Surg Endosc 18:1778, 2004.
32. Byron JW, Markenson G, Miyazawa K: A randomized comparison of Veress needle and direct trocar insertion for laparoscopy. Surg Gynecol Obstet 177:259, 1993.
33. Nezhat FR, Sifen SL, Evans D, Nezhat C: Comparison of direct insertion of disposable and standard reusable laparoscopic trocars and previous pneumoperitoneum with Veress needle. Obstet Gynecol 78:148, 1991.

Insufflation and the Pneumoperitoneum

34. Wolf JS, Stoller ML: The physiology of laparoscopy: Basic principles, complications and other considerations. J Urol 152:294, 1994.
35. Maunder RJ, Pierson DJ, Hudson LD: Subcutaneous and mediastinal emphysema: Pathophysiology, diagnosis and management. Arch Intern Med 144:1447, 1984.
36. Cooley JC, Gillespie JB: Mediastinal emphysema: Pathogenesis and management. Chest 49:104, 1966.
37. Venkatesh R, Kibel AS, Lee D, et al: Rapid resolution of carbon dioxide pneumothorax (capno-thorax) resulting from diaphragmatic injury during laparoscopic nephrectomy. J Urol 167:1387, 2002.

38. Abreu SC, Sharp DS, Ramani AP, et al: Thoracic complications during urological laparoscopy. J Urol 171:1451, 2004.

39. Joris JL, Chiche JD, Lamy ML: Pneumothorax during laparoscopic fundoplication: Diagnosis and treatment with positive end-expiratory pressure. Anesth Analg 81:993, 1995.

40. Carmichael DE: Laparoscopy: Cardiac considerations. Fertil Steril 22:69, 1971.

41. Morison DE, Riggs JRA: Cardiovascular collapse in laparoscopy. Can Med Assoc J 111:433, 1974.

42. Ostman PL, Pantle-Fisher FH, Faure EA, Glosten B: Circulatory collapse during laparoscopy. J Clin Anesth 2:129, 1990.

43. Bonjer HJ, Hazebroek EJ, Kazemier G, et al: Open versus closed establishment of pneumoperitoneum in laparoscopic surgery. Br J Surg 84:599, 1997.

44. Wolf JS, Stoller ML: The physiology of laparoscopy: Basic principles, complications, and other considerations. J Urol 152:294, 1994.

45. Gomar C, Fernandez C, Villalonga A, Nalda MA: Carbon dioxide embolism during laparoscopy and hysteroscopy. Ann Fr Anesth Reanim 4:380, 1985.

46. Shulum D, Aronson HB: Capnography in the early diagnosis of carbon dioxide embolism during laparoscopy. Can J Anaesth 31:455, 1984.

47. De Plater RMH, Jones ISC: Non-fatal carbon dioxide embolism during laparoscopy. Anaesth Intensive Care 17:359, 1989.

Vascular Injury

48. Parsons JK, Varkarakis I, Rha KH, et al: Complications of abdominal urologic laparoscopy: Longitudinal five-year analysis. Urology 63:27, 2004.

49. Chan D, Bishoff JT, Ratner L, et al: Endovascular gastrointestinal stapler device malfunction during laparoscopic nephrectomy: Early recognition and management. J Urol 164:319, 2000.

Gastrointestinal Injury

50. Parsons JK, Varkarakis I, Rha KH, et al: Complications of abdominal urologic laparoscopy: Longitudinal five-year analysis. Urology 63:27, 2004.

51. Reich H: Laparoscopic bowel injury. Surg Laparosc Endosc 2:74, 1992.

52. Bishoff JT, Allaf ME, Kirkels W, et al: Laparoscopic bowel injury: Incidence and clinical presentation. J Urol 161:887, 1999.

Pleural/Diaphragmatic Injury

53. Del Pizzo JJ, Jacobs SC, Bishoff JT, et al: Pleural injury during laparoscopic renal surgery: Early recognition and management. J Urol 169:41, 2003.

54. Potter SR, Kavoussi LR, Jackman SV: Management of diaphragmatic injury during laparoscopic nephrectomy. J Urol 165:1203, 2001.

Partial Nephrectomy

55. Ramani AP, Desai MM, Steinberg AP, et al: Complications of laparoscopic partial nephrectomy in 200 cases. J Urol 173:42, 2005.

56. Rassweiler JJ, Abbou C, Janetschek G, Jeschke K: Laparoscopic partial nephrectomy. The European Experience. Urol Clin North Am 27:721, 2000.

57. Kim FJ, Rha KH, Hernandez F, et al: Laparoscopic radical versus partial nephrectomy: Assessment of complications. J Urol 170:408, 2003.

58. Link RE, Bhayani SB, Allaf ME, et al: Exploring the learning curve, pathological outcomes and perioperative morbidity of laparoscopic partial nephrectomy performed for renal mass. J Urol 173:1690, 2005.

59. Guillonneau B, Bermudez H, Gholami H, et al: Laparoscopic partial nephrectomy for renal tumor: Single center experience comparing clamping and no clamping techniques of the renal vasculature. J Urol 169:483, 2003.

60. Gill IS, Ramani AP, Spaliviero M, et al: Improved hemostasis during laparoscopic partial nephrectomy using gelatin matrix thrombin sealant. Urology 65:463, 2005.

61. Campbell SC, Novick AC, Streem SB, et al: Complications of nephron sparing surgery for renal tumors. J Urol 151:1177, 1994.

62. Belldegrun A, Tsui KH, deKernion JB, Smith RB: Efficacy of nephron-sparing surgery for renal cell carcinoma: Analysis based on the new 1997 tumor-node-metastasis staging system. J Clin Oncol 17:2868, 1999.

63. Polascik TJ, Pound CR, Meng, et al: Partial nephrectomy: Technique, complications and pathological findings. J Urol 154:1312, 1995.

64. Bove P, Bhayani SB, Rha K, et al: Necessity of ureteral catheter during laparoscopic partial nephrectomy. J Urol 172:458, 2004.

65. Jeschke K, Peschel R, Wakonig J, et al: Laparoscopic nephron-sparing surgery for renal tumors. Urology 58:688, 2001.

Miscellaneous

66. Hashizume M, Sugimachi K: Study Group of Endoscopic Surgery in Kyushu Japan. Needle and trocar injury during laparoscopic surgery in Japan. Surg Endosc 11:1198, 1997.

67. Terranova SA, Siddiqui KM, Preminger GM, Albala DM: Hand-assisted laparoscopic renal surgery: Hand-port incision complications. J Endourol 18:775, 2004.

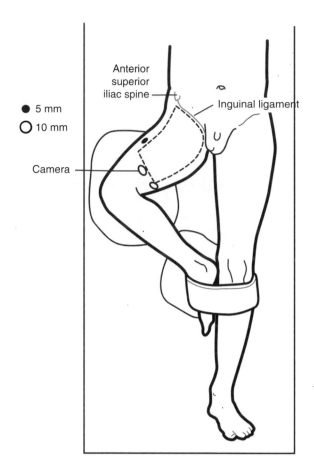

FIGURE 29-2. The patient is placed in a supine position, with the ipsilateral knee flexed and hip abducted. The foot on the side of dissection is secured to the contralateral leg in a unilateral dissection or both feet secured together in the case of a bilateral procedure. A pad placed under the bent knee will help maintain the correct position during the case.

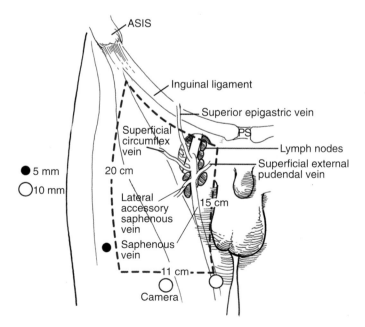

FIGURE 29-3. The limits of dissection are drawn on the skin. A line is drawn from the pubic tubercle to the anterior superior iliac crest. The width of the area of dissection is approximately 11 to 12 cm and the length 15 cm down the medial thigh and 20 cm on the lateral thigh. ASIS, anterior superior iliac spine.

Trocar placement is the same for the left and right sides. Place the trocars just outside the delineated area of dissection. Initially, place a 2.5-cm incision over the saphenous vein 15 cm below the pubic tubercle. Avoid making the incision any larger than 2.5 cm in order to prevent CO_2 escape during the procedure once the trocar is inserted and the subcutaneous cavity insufflated. Use sharp, fine scissors to develop the plane of dissection, elevating the skin from the deep membranous fascia and Scarpa's fascia toward the area of dissection drawn on the skin for as far as can be seen inside the lighted cavity. The laparoscope provides an excellent light source for the initial dissection. Place a Blunt Tip Trocar in the incision to create an airtight seal (U.S. Surgical, Norwalk, CT). The Blunt Tip Trocar is ideal for this procedure because its unique internal balloon and foam collar create an excellent seal and leave a very small profile inside the area of dissection. This trocar will become the medial working trocar, and because it is 10 mm, it can accommodate a retrieval bag to remove lymph node packets during the procedure. If a large nodal packet is placed in the bag and cannot be extracted through the trocar, the balloon on the trocar can be deflated and the packet (secured inside the retrieval bag) can be extracted directly through the incision. To prevent seeding the trocar site, do not extract fatty and lymphatic tissue specimens directly through the skin incision without placing them inside an extraction bag.

Place a second 2.5-cm incision outside the area of dissection approximately 16 cm inferior to the middle of the inguinal ligament. Use scissors to establish the correct plane of dissection toward the first trocar until the two planes of dissection are joined and a second Blunt Tip Trocar is placed. The laparoscope is usually placed through the second trocar during the procedure. Insufflate the working space to a pressure of 5 mm Hg.

Use a pair of endoscopic scissors or ultrasonic shears to dissect the inferior skin margin toward the edge of the surgical field so that the third trocar can be placed. Place a 5-mm threaded trocar outside the area of dissection approximately 15 cm below the iliac crest (Fig. 29–4).

PROCEDURE

Divide inguinal lymph nodes into superficial and deep nodes. The superficial nodes are those located anterior to the fascia lata and the deep nodes posterior to the fascia lata. Carry the inguinal lymph nodes dissection 2 cm above the inguinal ligament superiorly, laterally to the sartorius muscle and medially to the adductor longus. The superficial nodes are located in four quadrants centered around the saphenofemoral junction:

1. In the area of the superficial circumflex iliac vein
2. In the area of the superficial epigastric vein and the superficial external pudendal vein
3. In the inferomedial quadrant around the saphenous vein
4. Around the insertion of the superficial circumflex iliac vein and the lateral accessory saphenous vein[5] (Fig. 29–5)

The deep inguinal lymph nodes include the most cephalad node known as the node of Cloquet located in the area of the femoral vein and the lacunar ligament (Fig. 29–6).

The dissection begins above Scarpa's fascia anteriorly removing the tissue located between the skin and the fascia lata. Early

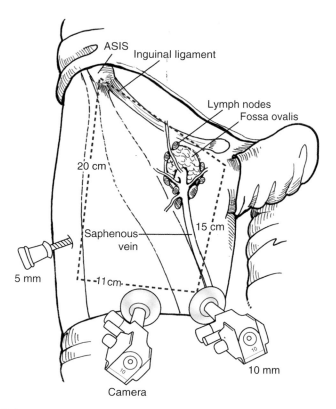

FIGURE 29–4. The trocars are placed just outside the delineated area of dissection. The first is placed approximately 15 cm below the pubic tubercle over the saphenous vein. A Blunt Tip Trocar is placed in the incision to create an airtight seal (Autosuture, U.S. Surgical, Norwalk, CT). A second 2.5-cm incision is placed outside the area of dissection approximately 16 cm inferior to the middle of the inguinal ligament, and a second Blunt Tip Trocar is placed. The laparoscope is usually placed through the second trocar during the procedure. A 5-mm threaded trocar is placed outside the area of dissection approximately 15 cm below the iliac crest.

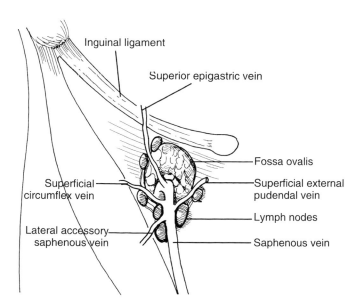

FIGURE 29–5. The superficial nodes are located in four quadrants centered around the saphenofemoral junction: (1) nodes in the area of the superficial circumflex iliac vein, (2) nodes in the area of the superficial epigastric vein and the superficial external pudendal vein, (3) nodes located in the inferomedial quadrant around the saphenous vein, and (4) nodes around the insertion of the superficial circumflex iliac vein and the lateral accessory saphenous vein.

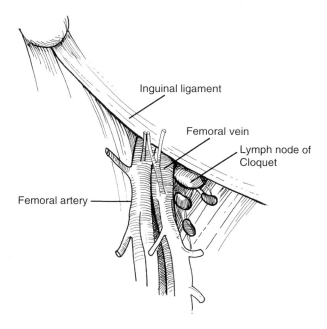

FIGURE 29–6. The deep inguinal lymph nodes are located under the fascia lata and include the most cephalad node known as the node of Cloquet located in the area of the femoral vein and the lacunar ligament.

in the dissection, identify and preserve the saphenous vein, if possible. It helps to identify the borders of dissection medially at the adductor longus and laterally at the sartorius muscle edges. In some patients, it can be difficult to identify these landmarks without opening the fascia lata, but the margins marked on the skin will help in the dissection of the superficial nodal tissue. Divide subcutaneous vessels and saphenous branches using ultrasonic energy or electrocautery. Dissect lymph node–bearing tissue from the fascia lata to the fossa ovalis.

As the dissection progresses toward the inguinal ligament, identify the external ring and remove the fat and lymphatics in the area of the cord to the base of the penis medially. Continue the lymph node dissection 3 to 4 cm superior to the inguinal ligament. Once the nodal tissue and fat are removed from the external oblique and the inguinal ligament, identify the femoral vessels inside the femoral sheath.

To gain access to the deep nodes, open the fascia lata to the edge of the adductor longus medially and the sartoris muscle laterally. Carefully remove the triangle-shaped lymph packet within the femoral triangle. Opening the femoral sheath down toward the apex of the triangle reveals the deep lymph nodes. Medial dissection frees the node of Cloquet. Remove any residual tissue between the femoral artery and vein. Take care to prevent injury to the femoral nerve by limiting the lateral dissection to the femoral artery.

If the skin overlying the exposed vessels seems compromised in any way, mobilize the sartorius from the anterior superior iliac crest using ultrasonic or bipolar cautery, and transfer it over the exposed vessels. Use three or four size 2-0 PDS sutures to attach the sartorius muscle to the inguinal ligament.

At the end of the procedure, place a 7-mm JP drain inside the cavity to ensure drainage at the most dependent site of dissection. Place this through either the 5-mm trocar site or a new site chosen as needed. Close the two 10-mm trocar sites with skin adhesive or subcuticular sutures. Once the skin adhesive